Supplementary
Prescribing
A Practical Guide

Published by Remedica
Commonwealth House, 1 New Oxford Street, London WC1A 1NU, UK
Civic Opera Building, 20 North Wacker Drive, Suite 1642, Chicago, IL 60606, USA

info@remedicabooks.com
www.remedicabooks.com
Tel: +44 20 7759 2999
Fax: +44 20 7759 2951

Publisher: Andrew Ward
In-house editors: Catherine Booth and Carolyn Dunn
Design and artwork: AS&K Skylight Creative Services

Remedica is a member of the AS&K Media Partnership.

ISBN-10: 1 901346 93 5
ISBN-13: 978 1 901346 93 0
British Library Cataloguing-in-Publication Data
A catalogue record for this book is available from the British Library.

Surviving Prescribing: A Practical Guide

Editors

Rob Shulman
ICU Clinical Pharmacist
University College London Hospitals
London

Hugh Montgomery
Consultant Intensivist
University College London Hospitals
London

Jane Ng
Neurosurgical Research Registrar
Department of Neuroscience
Charing Cross Hospital
London

Simon Keady
Women's and Children Lead Pharmacist
University College London Hospitals
London

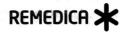

REMEDICA ✱

Contributors

Suparna Bali
Lead Surgical Pharmacist,
Royal Free Hospital, London, UK

David Brull
Consultant Cardiologist,
Whittington Hospital, London, UK

Bridget Coleman
Medicines Management Pharmacist,
Whittington Hospital, London, UK

Evelyn Frank
Senior Pharmacist,
National Hospital for Neurology
and Neurosurgery, London, UK

Caroline Green
Specialist Registrar, Gastroenterology,
Oxford Radcliffe Hospitals, Oxford, UK

Anthony Grosso
Principal Pharmacist, Drug Usage
& Formulary Management,
University College London Hospitals,
London, UK

Olivia Hameer
GI and Surgical Pharmacist,
University College London Hospitals,
London, UK

Yogini Jani
Formerly Senior Clinical Pharmacist,
University College London Hospitals,
London, UK

Dipty Joshi
Renal Clinical Pharmacist,
University College London Hospitals,
London, UK

Simon Keady
Women's and Children
Lead Pharmacist,
University College London Hospitals,
London, UK

Roman Landowski
Senior Pharmacist,
Medicines Information
University College London Hospitals,
London, UK

Fiona Maguire
Women's Services
Clinical Pharmacist,
University College London
Hospitals, London, UK

Nicola Mayne
Adolescent/Paediatric
Clinical Pharmacist,
University College London
Hospitals, London, UK

Hugh Montgomery
Consultant Intensivist,
University College London
Hospitals, London, UK

Jane Ng
Neurosurgical Research Registrar,
Department of Neuroscience,
Charing Cross Hospital, London

Simon Noble
Senior Lecturer and Honorary
Consultant, Cardiff University;
Royal Gwent Hospital, Cardiff, UK

Preet Panesar
Formerly Medicine and Emergency
Services/Diabetes Pharmacist,
University College London
Hospitals, London, UK

Rob Shulman
ICU Clinical Pharmacist,
University College London
Hospitals, London, UK

Claire Turner
Specialist Registrar in Palliative
Medicine, Ty Olwen, Swansea, UK

Rebecca White
Lead Pharmacist,
Surgery & Nutrition,
Oxford Radcliffe Hospitals,
Oxford, UK

Peter Wilson
Consultant Microbiologist,
University College London
Hospitals, London, UK

Preface

Whether you are a doctor, nurse or pharmacist, it is very likely that you will be involved in prescribing drugs or in making the safest and most effective use of medicines. As a student in any of these disciplines, you are also expected to at least understand the practical issues relating to drug use.

All of you will recognise how easy it is to cause a patient harm. And you will also know how hard it is to find helpful information. We are all taught the basics of drug absorption, distribution and interaction, and hospital formularies (and reference texts such as the *BNF*) are often excellent resources for drug doses and the like.

But what about the practical stuff?

- We all know that antibiotics can interact with warfarin in a dangerous way, but how are you meant to adjust the doses? And what about restarting warfarin after surgery?

- You're treating a patient suffering from alcohol withdrawal… what regimens are available to you?

- How do you manage 'patient-controlled analgesia'?

- How do you manage a paracetamol overdose when you don't know the time of paracetamol ingestion?

This book will tell you.

Written by clinical pharmacists and doctors with years of experience, this collection of handy hints, tips and protocols will help you to prescribe simply, safely and with confidence.

Use it as a textbook. Use it as a reference on the ward or in the clinic. But most of all, do use it… and enjoy it, too.

Contents

Abbreviations   viii
The Basics of Safe Drug Use   x

Section 1: Prescribing for Patient Groups   1

1.	Prescribing in Pregnancy	3
2.	Prescribing in Breastfeeding	11
3.	Prescribing in Children	15
4.	Prescribing in Older Patients	20
5.	Prescribing in Renal Disease	23
6.	Treating Diabetes	34
7.	Management of the Acutely Confused Patient	40
8.	Alcohol Dependence and the DTs	43

Section 2: Emergency Prescribing   49

1.	Diabetic Ketoacidosis	51
2.	Hyperosmolar Non-ketotic Coma	53
3.	Hypoglycaemia	55
4.	Paracetamol Overdose	57
5.	Emergency Prescribing in Cardiology	60
6.	Emergency Prescribing in Neurosurgery	68
7.	Massive Pulmonary Embolism	73
8.	Electrolyte and Metabolic Emergencies	75
9.	Respiratory Emergencies	82

Section 3: Gastrointestinal System   87

1.	Practical Prescribing in General Gastroenterology	89
2.	Constipation in the Adult Patient	92
3.	Nausea and Vomiting	95
4.	Safe Prescribing in Liver Disease	97
5.	Practical Total Parenteral Nutrition	99

Section 4: Central Nervous System 103

1. Analgesia   105
2. Patient-controlled Analgesia   114
3. Epidural Analgesia   117
4. Prescribing in Palliative Care   121
5. Fit for a Fit: Adults with Seizures   126
6. Insomnia   131

Section 5: Blood 137

1. Warfarin Prescribing   139
2. Parenteral Anti-coagulation   146

Section 6: Surgery 153

1. Practical Prescribing in the Surgical Patient   155
2. Diabetes and Surgery   163
3. Bowel Preparation   166

Section 7: Miscellaneous 169

1. Calculations for the Prescriber   171
2. Corticosteroids   176
3. Infections   179
4. Therapeutic Drug Monitoring   192
5. Drug Hypersensitivities and Contraindications 204
6. Interactions that Matter   209
7. Intravenous Therapy   218

Index 221

Abbreviations

ACE	angiotensin-converting enzyme
ACS	acute coronary syndromes
AF	atrial fibrillation
APTT	activated partial thromboplastin time
ARB	angiotensin receptor blocker
ARF	acute renal failure
AV	atrioventricular
BD	twice a day
BNF	British National Formulary
BP	blood pressure
CBW	corrected body weight
COPD	chronic obstructive pulmonary disease
COX	cyclooxygenase
CPR	cardiopulmonary resuscitation
CSM	Committee on Safety of Medicines
CT	computed tomography
DC	direct current
DKA	diabetic ketoacidosis
DT	delirium tremens
DVT	deep venous thrombosis
EBW	excess body weight
ECG	electrocardiogram
FBC	full blood count
FFP	fresh-frozen plasma
GFR	glomerular filtration rate
GI	gastrointestinal
GIK	glucose–insulin–potassium
HDU	high-dependency unit
IBW	ideal body weight
ICP	intracranial pressure
ICU	intensive care unit
IM	intramuscular
INR	international normalisation ratio

IV	intravenous
LFT	liver function test
LMWH	low molecular weight heparin
MCV	mean cell volume
MI	myocardial infarction
MRSA	methicillin-resistant *Staphylococcus aureus*
NAC	N-acetylcysteine
NBM	nil by mouth
NG	nasogastric
NICE	National Institute for Clinical Excellence
NSAID	non-steroidal anti-inflammatory drug
OD	once a day
ON	once a night
PE	pulmonary embolism
PO	by mouth
PPI	proton-pump inhibitor
PR	by rectum
PRN	as needed
QDS	four times a day
S/L	sublingual
SAH	subarachnoid haemorrhage
SC	subcutaneous
SSRI	selective serotonin reuptake inhibitor
TDM	therapeutic blood monitoring
TDS	three times a day
U&Es	urea and electrolytes
UTI	urinary tract infection

The Basics of Safe Drug Use

Here, 'safe drug use' refers to your prescription and administration, not recreational use. In this regard, there are a few 'golden rules' that will keep you out of trouble (and court!).

Ready?

You can't be expected to 'know it all' let alone remember it all. So seek references!

- Find *local policies/protocols* in your hospital formulary and use them.

- *Check the BNF* when in doubt. It's now available on-line, too. As well as dosing, it will tell you indications, contraindications, interactions, side effects, use in hepatic and renal failure and use in pregnancy. It also includes NICE guidelines, other disease management guidelines (eg, British Thoracic Society guidelines on acute asthma) and CSM warnings.

- *Ask your pharmacy* for help as a matter of routine, not just when *"It's all gone wrong!"*

Steady...

Whether your hospital uses a paper chart or a funky electronic system, it will have separate prescribing sections. These include sections for one-off 'stat' doses of drugs, regular medications, as-required 'PRN' drugs, infusions and IV fluids. There might also be supplementary charts for 'specialist' items (eg, total parenteral nutrition, anti-coagulation, chemotherapy). *Be careful of where you write your prescription!* If incorrectly done, it can mean your patient doesn't get the drug or you end up correcting lots of charts.

GO!

You have now decided what to prescribe and at what dose, and have chosen where to write the prescription. Now use these *SICKL*y tips to avoid mistakes:

Simplify

* *Try not to give drugs at all!* All drugs have side effects and are hazardous. Every now and then, the drug you give will contribute (directly or indirectly) to a death.

* *Do you really have to give it?* Will the green spit or sore throat not get better on its own? Is the cough so bad that codeine linctus and its side effects of constipation and drowsiness are worth it? Can you do anything without drugs (eg, reassurance, ear plugs if noise is keeping a patient awake, fruit and coffee for constipation)?

* Try to *cross off a drug* every time you review a chart.

* Wherever possible, *seek the 'once-a-day' drug* from a class. Compliance will be better on discharge and the fewer 'prescribing events', the fewer things that can go wrong!

Interrogate your patient and their chart

* *Are all their allergies documented?* And what does the patient mean by 'allergy' to toxocillin? That they got a runny nose, a rash or full-blown anaphylaxis? Are you about to prescribe a drug that will make their skin peel off?

* *What is your patient's weight?* You need to know this to prescribe certain drugs (eg, LMWH and once-daily gentamicin).

- *What is your patient's height?* This is needed to calculate surface area and ideal/excess body weight, which are required for gentamicin dosing and chemotherapeutics. Importantly, has the patient's weight changed significantly since the drug was prescribed, thus changing the prescribed dose?

Clarify

- Be clear in *writing* a prescription. Do not rush. Is there *any* chance that your script will be misread?

- Be clear in *reasoning*. Add comments where needed (eg, "Patient has been on sleepazepam for 20 years and withdraws without it – please give").

- Be clear in *timing* – in particular, start and stop times. Cross off the chart when you want the course to be changed. Write up the reducing doses for a full course, so that when you are next doing 'days' 5 weeks on, you don't find the patient still on 60 mg prednisolone!

Check

- Check *doses*, etc. of unfamiliar drugs before prescribing.

- Check for *interactions* with the other charted drugs.

- If you are administering, check that the doctor was *correct* in what they wrote.

- Check everything that you do at least twice. With IV drugs, *never* be lazy. When you're tired, you can read what you expect to see. Always ask someone else to check the ampoule!

Know

Have a basic understanding of the class of drug you are giving. Know a line or two about how it works. This is your safety lock: it allows you to hear alarm bells, nudging you to recall a drug interaction or side effect. Back this up by revising, from time to time, the basic side effects and interactions of a drug and its class.

Think *Levels*!

Consider factors that might alter drug levels (eg, age, disease, other drugs). Does the drug you are about to prescribe need its levels monitored? Are you sure? Check. Call the pharmacy. Call microbiology. Call a colleague. But *do call!* When you're sure, be clear about when levels should be taken, and how often. And ensure that they are taken and acted upon. Put some fail-safes in – mark the chart: "Not to be given until dr has reviewed levels" or "Do not give until INR has been seen."

And, lastly, think who will continue to review the patient's levels when they are discharged? Have you booked them into an anti-coagulant clinic?

TOP TIPS: SICKLy

So, familiarise yourself with the chart and back yourself up with some information. Then, think:

- *S*implify the chart (fewer drugs, fewer doses).

- *I*nterrogate the notes/chart/patient for allergies and interactions.

- *C*larify your chart. Be clear with your writing, reasoning and timing.

- *C*heck doses, interactions and all ampoules.

- *K*now your drug classes, their mechanisms and major side effects/interactions.

- *L*evels: think about factors that alter levels, and the need for monitoring them.

Finally, congratulations! Your patient has survived! Now safely discharge them!

- Note the patient's discharge medications carefully, following the rules above.

- Clearly mark any changes from their admission medications, and include the reasons for these changes.

- Ensure that the patient is aware of these changes – drugs only work if the patient actually takes them.

- Organise any necessary follow-up (eg, repeat phenytoin or INR levels, GP appointment after completion of steroid reduction for acute asthma).

Hugh Montgomery, Yogini Jani and Jane Ng

1

Prescribing for Patient Groups

1. Prescribing in Pregnancy	3
2. Prescribing in Breastfeeding	11
3. Prescribing in Children	15
4. Prescribing in Older Patients	20
5. Prescribing in Renal Disease	23
6. Treating Diabetes	34
7. Management of the Acutely Confused Patient	40
8. Alcohol Dependence and the DTs	43

Prescribing in Pregnancy

Roman Landowski

The thalidomide disaster of 1958–1962 showed that drugs *do* reach the foetus and *can* cause harm. Even now, of the 2–3% of children born in the UK with a recognised birth defect, drugs (illicit or prescription) are still implicated in 1–2%. *Think before prescribing!*

Weighing the risks

Around 10–20 drugs have been 'proven' safe in pregnancy. A similar number of related drugs are assumed to be so. A further similar number have been 'proven' dangerous to the foetus. But, for the majority, there is no proof of safety or danger. The advice of manufacturers not to prescribe in pregnancy unless the benefit outweighs the risk is pretty useless when the risk isn't quantified!

So what can be done in practice?

Think of the possible *benefit* to the mother

- Consider the danger of the condition. Are we talking threadworms or thrombosis, heart attack or heartburn? In other words, what is the risk of *not* treating?

- How effective is the drug likely to be? If the condition is not dangerous and the benefits of treatment are minor, are there any non-drug measures that might help (eg, finger hygiene for 6 weeks to break a threadworm lifecycle? Regular snacks for heartburn?)

- Will the foetus be at risk if you don't treat the disease? This is the conundrum that you face when an epileptic tells you that she is pregnant – both the disease and its treatments are known to have adverse effects on the foetus.

Then, think of the *risk* to the foetus

Most of the time, you don't know the risk to the foetus. But, you do know that the risk is likely to change with the trimester. Drugs can be safe in one trimester and dangerous in another.

Pre-embryonic period

Drugs taken in the first 17 days after conception exert an 'all or nothing' effect. The cluster of cells is either completely killed off, which results in a late menstrual bleed (and the woman most likely never realises she was pregnant), or the cells recover completely and develop normally. If exposure is confined to this period and the woman finds herself still pregnant then you can be confident that the drug has had no effect on the foetus.

First trimester

The period of organ formation. This period holds the greatest risk of drug-induced teratogenesis (eg, spina bifida is caused by exposure to anti-folate drugs such as trimethoprim at this time). Try to delay all drugs until the second trimester.

Second and third trimesters

The organs are developing and maturing. Drugs will affect their function rather than their structure (eg, enalapril can cause foetal renal failure with exposure at this time).

Exposure near term risks labour, perinatal and neonatal complications. Neonatal respiratory depression is a feature of pethidine administration during labour.

Then, think *form* of administration

Topical drugs penetrate the placenta less – so reach for clotrimazole rather than fluconazole when treating thrush.

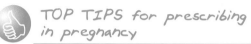 **TOP TIPS for prescribing in pregnancy**

The rules governing prescribing in pregnancy can be summarised as *Best Think First*!

- **Best** Benefit – are the benefits of treatment obvious and necessary? Or not?

- **Think** Trimester – are there safer drugs at this stage of pregnancy?

- **First** Form – are topical or minimally absorbed preparations available?

Then, remember siCkly – Check! Check written sources. Check with your registrar. Check with your pharmacist. Appendix 4 of the *BNF* is brief and mentions all of the recognised problem drugs, but lacks detail where the situation is less cut and dried.

And, of course, *never take chances*. If you're unsure, ring the medicines information centre in your local hospital pharmacy and ask! Your defence organisation will thank you!

Common prescriptions

Analgesics

- Paracetamol is safe in all stages of pregnancy.

- Opioids such as dihydrocodeine, morphine and methadone do not cause birth defects. However, if they are used throughout pregnancy then the neonate can experience a distressing withdrawal syndrome. Due to the risk of fitting, this is best managed on a neonatal unit.

- NSAIDs such as ibuprofen or diclofenac can cause premature closure of the ductus arteriosus (leading to pulmonary hypertension) if used in late pregnancy. They can also cause an increase in maternal blood loss during labour due to their anti-platelet effects.

Anti-asthmatics

- Inhaled medicines are safe because they don't achieve significant blood levels. This includes salbutamol – when given systemically salbutamol relaxes the uterine muscle, but when inhaled it does not prolong labour.

- Systemic steroids (eg, prednisolone) can increase the risk of cleft lip and cleft palate if used in the first trimester, so keep courses short. High-dose inhaled steroids (eg, beclomethasone 1,500 µg/day) theoretically carry the same risk.

Antibiotics

- Penicillins (eg, amoxicillin, flucloxacillin) and cephalosporins (eg, cefuroxime, cefalexin) are considered to be safe.

- Quinolones such as ciprofloxacin have caused foetal arthropathy in animal studies, but very rarely in humans. Nevertheless, they should be avoided where possible.

- Trimethoprim is an anti-folate drug that has been associated with an increase in birth defects following first trimester exposure.

- Tetracyclines (eg, doxycycline, oxytetracycline) cause permanent yellow–brown bands to appear on the teeth following exposure from about 24 weeks' gestation.

Anti-coagulants

- LMWHs are the safest as they do not cross the placenta. Some (eg, dalteparin) have positive evidence for safety in pregnancy.

- Unfractionated heparin is safe for the foetus, but can cause maternal osteoporosis if used for >6 months in pregnancy.

- Warfarin has been associated with foetal intracranial bleeds when used in the second and third trimesters, which might lead to *in utero* death. Foetal warfarin syndrome has also been described following exposure between gestational weeks 6–9. This includes nasal, ocular, ear, cardiac, skeletal and mental defects.

Anti-emetics

- Anti-histamines such as cyclizine and promethazine are the drugs of choice. They have been around for ages without evidence of harm.

- Prochlorperazine is also considered safe for the foetus, but young women are at increased risk of experiencing dose-related extrapyramidal side effects.

Anti-convulsants

- Carbamazepine and valproate are associated with neural tube defects (eg, spina bifida, anencephaly) when given in the first trimester. To counter this, folic acid 5 mg/day should be co-prescribed throughout pregnancy.

- Carbamazepine, phenytoin and phenobarbitone all induce the metabolism of vitamin K, so it is common to co-prescribe phytomenadione 20 mg OD for the last month of pregnancy to reduce the chance of haemorrhagic disease of the newborn.

Foetal anti-epileptic syndrome refers to a range of somatic defects associated with the drugs mentioned above. It includes cleft lip, cleft palate, hypertelorism, low-set ears, retrognathia and shortened distal phalanges. There is also some evidence that these drugs slow mental development in childhood, whilst a withdrawal reaction (agitation) has been seen in neonates exposed to phenobarbitone and benzodiazepines such as clonazepam. The risks of defects can be lowered by reducing the number of anti-epileptic drugs and the doses used.

Anti-fungals

- There is sufficient experience with clotrimazole cream and pessaries to assume that these are safe.

- Avoid fluconazole in the first trimester as high doses (≥400 mg/day) have been associated with craniofacial and skeletal defects similar to Antley–Bixler syndrome.

Anti-hypertensives

- Methyldopa and hydralazine are considered to be safe, mainly because they have been around for a long time without any obvious problems cropping up.

- Beta-blockers are associated with intrauterine growth retardation due to placental vasoconstriction, although this is less likely with the vasodilatory labetalol. This effect is most noticeable after exposure in the second and third trimesters. Beta-blockers at term can also cause neonatal bradycardia and hypoglycaemia.

- ACE inhibitors are known to reduce foetal renal function when prescribed in the second and third trimesters. Oligohydramnios ensues, which can lead to pulmonary hypoplasia and skeletal defects.

- ARBs (eg, losartan, irbesartan) have similar pharmacological effects as ACE inhibitors, so are assumed to carry the same risks.

Gastroprotective agents

- There are reasonable data to assume that ranitidine and omeprazole are not major teratogens.

- Misoprostol is a uterine stimulant that causes uterine contractions. It can be used in high single doses

(800 µg) for termination of pregnancy. There is a risk of miscarriage if it is used at any stage of pregnancy.

Laxatives

- Senna is licensed, so is as safe as drugs in pregnancy get. The glycerin suppositories lactulose and ispaghula work locally and have minimal systemic absorption, so are also safe.

- Castor oil is such a strong purgative that it has been used to induce uterine contractions. It can cause miscarriage and should be avoided.

Psychiatric drugs

- Tricyclic anti-depressants (eg, amitriptyline, lofepramine) are not associated with birth defects, but might cause an increased risk of miscarriage.

- SSRIs may increase the risk of cardiac septal defects in the first trimester and persistent pulmonary hypertension of the newborn if used after week 20 of pregnancy.

- Neonatal withdrawal syndrome (insomnia, crying, poor feeding) is possible in infants exposed *in utero* during the last few months of pregnancy. This is particularly an issue with paroxetine, where cases of hypoglycaemia have also been seen.

- Lithium increases the risk of Ebstein's anomaly. This heart valve defect is seen far more frequently in children exposed to lithium, but the absolute incidence is still very low (probably <1%).

- Temazepam is safe when used alone, although it can lead to neonatal withdrawal. However, it has caused *in utero* death when taken with diphenhydramine, which is present in several over-the-counter preparations (eg, Nytol®, Benylin 4-Flu®).

Skin diseases

- Topical creams are all safe, including topical isotretinoin. Unfortunately, oral isotretinoin is the most notorious teratogen with a current UK product licence, so both patients and prescribers are naturally reluctant to use its topical cousin.

- Isotretinoin capsules cause defects in about one third of children who are exposed during the first trimester. There is a recognised pattern of defects involving cardiac and craniofacial abnormalities. Acitretin, another vitamin A analogue, carries the same risks as excess vitamin A in pregnancy. Yes, young girls are sensitive about their looks and, yes, acne causes a lot of teenage angst, but it's never bad enough to warrant isotretinoin if she's pregnant!

- First trimester use of prednisolone and other systemic steroids might increase the risk of cleft lip and cleft palate, so use topical steroids or keep systemic courses short. Topical steroids carry the same kind of risks as systemic steroids, but are safer because you just don't absorb that much. For example, a pregnant woman who uses one 30 g tube of betnovate a week would only be exposing her foetus to the equivalent of 17 mg hydrocortisone a day, which, being physiological, is unlikely to cause problems.

Prescribing in Breastfeeding

2

Fiona Maguire

Here is a very brief guide to get you through the on-call. This is a very specialist field, where the evidence base is far from exhaustive. Check with your registrar/consultant and pharmacist! Make sure that you know something about the drugs you are prescribing – does anything raise alarm bells?

The rules

Rule 1. Remember *S*ickly – keep it *S*imple. Don't ever prescribe unless absolutely necessary. Most mums will happily put up with a headache rather than take paracetamol. However, there are some cases where drugs must be given and breastfeeding is contraindicated (eg, in those taking anti-cancer agents).

Rule 2. Select the class of drug that you want to use. Now select the drug with the shortest half-life, the most evidence-based information and the smallest number of side effects.

Rule 3. Look for drugs with once-daily administration. This gives the mother the option to feed or express when levels of the drug are at their lowest.

Rule 4. Ask yourself:

- How much drug is getting into the milk?
- What are the associated risks to the infant?

The *BNF* is insufficient, so also ask your pharmacist/medicines information centre.

Rule 5. Tell the parents what side effects to look out for. Whilst the vast majority of antibiotics are safe in breastfeeding, they *will* cross into the milk. The parents can expect an increase in their nappy bill.

Rule 6. If a treatment decreases the amount of breast milk being produced (eg, diuretics), recommend more visits to the breast rather than topping up with infant formula. Explain to the mother that this needs to be balanced against an increased risk of nipple soreness.

Rule 7. If the mother has to stop breastfeeding during a short course of treatment, advise her to express and discard.

Understanding the literature

Drugs are often classified in the following manner:

"Compatible with breastfeeding."
Enough said.

"Compatible with breastfeeding. Monitor infant for side effects."
The drug can theoretically cause side effects, but these have either not been seen before or are minor in nature. Reassure the parents, explain what to look out for and ask the mother to return if she has any concerns.

"Avoid if possible. Monitor infant for side effects."
Often the drug has been reported to cause a serious side effect. It should only be used if absolutely necessary and where there is no other treatment available. Arrange regular follow-ups to support monitoring. A decision might need to be taken to stop therapy.

"Avoid if possible. May inhibit lactation."
Try to avoid these drugs, especially if taking them will have a negative impact upon the mother's psychological wellbeing. Reduced lactation can be countered by regular trips to the breast.

"Avoid."
If this is the only option for treatment, seek specialist help. The issues of not breastfeeding need to be explained, and other people will have had more experience in this than you.

'Safe' drugs

Drugs that are safe to give in normal adult doses to the mother of a normal term infant include:

- Antibiotics – penicillins, cephalosporins, erythromycin (and gentamicin, provided that you have understood our chapter on *Therapeutic drug monitoring* – **Section 7, Chapter 4**).

- NSAIDs – diclofenac and ibuprofen are the drugs of choice.

- Asthma therapy – all inhalers, theophylline.

- Non-sedating anti-histamines – eg, cetirizine.

- Corticosteroids – lower doses of short courses of prednisolone (eg, ≤30 mg daily).

- Beta-blockers – labetalol is the drug of choice. Most other beta-blockers will pass into the milk and cause all sorts of side effects in the child, including bradycardia and hypotension.

- Laxatives – senna, lactulose and ispaghula are suitable as they are not absorbed from the GI tract. Avoid co-danthramer.

- LMWHs – dalteparin and enoxaparin are safe.

Caution required

Drugs to be used with caution (ie, use minimum dose possible) include:

- Opioid analgesics and anti-psychotics – warn the mother to look out for sedation and to stop breastfeeding if her child becomes very sleepy. Avoid high doses and avoid lithium.

- Anti-convulsants – sodium valproate and carbamazepine. Other anti-convulsants might need to be used in exceptional circumstances because of the needs of the mother. The baby will need to be monitored, and there are few published data.

- Anti-depressants – eg, non-sedating tricyclics and SSRIs are used in post-natal depression. Risk–benefit analysis usually favours prescribing, but watch out for growth problems and withdrawal. There might also be developmental problems.

Avoid if possible

Avoid breastfeeding if at all possible (and discuss with consultant) with:

- drugs of abuse

- high-dose sedative drugs

- immunosuppressants

Always avoid

Drugs that should always lead the patient to avoid breastfeeding include:

- cytotoxic agents

- radioactive substances

Prescribing in Children

3

Simon Keady

Definitions of age groups

Neonate: birth to 1 month.
Infant: 1 month to 2 years.
Child: 2–12 years.
Adolescent: 12–18 years.

General principles of prescribing

When it comes to prescribing, children are not 'little adults'.

- Some adult drugs are banned in children.

- Drug doses often don't just 'scale down' by weight.

- Many products contain excipients that are risky for kids, eg, alcohol (phenobarbitone, ranitidine, senna), propylene glycol (pyridoxine injection) and dyes.

- Growing teeth rot easily: sugar-free formulations should be used wherever possible or, if not possible, the child should brush their teeth after each dose.

- Other sweetening agents have their own problems: large amounts of sorbitol cause diarrhoea, whilst aspartame contains phenylalanine so must be used with caution in patients with phenylketonuria.

In addition, many drugs prescribed in children are 'off label' or unlicensed, for a variety of reasons (more on this below). You are allowed to do this, as long as you have taken the responsibility to personally ensure that you have adequate information to support the quality, efficacy, safety and use of the drug prior to prescribing. If you're not sure, ask. Don't leave it until the last minute.

Examples of why a drug might be unlicensed include:

- Only just undergoing clinical trials in adults.

- Prepared extemporaneously.

- Imported from another country.

- Manufactured under a special manufacturing licence.

- The product is not a medicine, but is being used to treat a rare condition.

The best advice, therefore, is that unless you are a paediatrician you should not be prescribing! If you have to prescribe, always check with a reputable paediatric formulary (eg, *BNF for Children*) and with locally agreed policies – and then with a paediatrician if you have any doubt *at all*.

The basic principles of prescribing in children are no different to those for adults (see *The basics of safe drug use*). However, given that this might be unfamiliar ground – and that incorrect dosing can be catastrophic – see our Top Tips for avoiding medication errors.

Routes of administration

When administering drugs to children, each route of administration has its advantages and disadvantages. The optimal routes should be chosen (see **Table 1**).

Table 1. Advantages and disadvantages of the different routes of drug administration in children.

Route	Advantages	Disadvantages
Intravenous	Predictable blood levels	Fragility of veins
		Risk of extravasation
Intramuscular	None	Painful
		Erratic absorption
Oral	Easiest	Lack of suitable dosage forms
	Convenient	Mixing with feeds
	Accurate administration with oral syringes	
Rectal	Rapid onset of action (eg, diazepam for fitting)	Lack of suitable dosage forms
		Erratic absorption (eg, theophylline)
Inhalation	Spacers can improve delivery of drug	Lack of coordination in young children
	Paediatric formularies will recommend suitable ones	

TOP TIPS for avoiding medication errors

- Always take care with calculations.

- Get someone to double-check your calculations if you're at all unsure.

- Prescribe in whole units – avoid decimal points (eg, 100 micrograms not 0.1 mg).

- When writing prescriptions, write the units out in full (eg, 'micrograms' not 'mcg' or 'µg').

- Never use a trailing zero (eg, 5 mg not 5.0 mg).

Concordance

Involve parents/carers and (if possible) the child from a very early stage. Both verbal and written information should be provided at a level that is easy to understand. Additional information is often required if patient information leaflets are provided from the manufacturer. These often state "Not recommended for use in children," which can cause additional alarm and confusion in parents. Involve your paediatric pharmacist in explaining the issues, as you can be certain that they will become involved when the patient is next admitted after not getting their medicine. This type of counselling is very important in optimising concordance.

 TOP TIPS for improving compliance in children

- Consider ease of administration.

- Tailor treatment to the child's daily routine.

- Set treatment goals in collaboration with the child, if possible.

- Provide suitable information to caregivers.

Common mistakes

Think volume!
Example: 'furosemide 5 mL TDS'. Formulations available are 1 mg/mL, 4 mg/mL, 8 mg/mL and 10 mg/mL – so the dose will vary each time... and overdose is possible.

Think decimals!
Example: it is easy to write morphine 20–40 mg, rather than 2–4 mg... and mistakes like this can kill.

Think 'non-adult' dose!

Example: if prescribing on a mg/kg basis, always ensure that you don't go over the recommended adult maximum, ie, prescribing 1.5 g paracetamol rather than the recommended ceiling of 1 g... which can cause liver failure and death.

Reporting adverse drug reactions

Little is known about the safe use of some medicines in children. Children are not usually exposed to medicines in clinical trials. It is important to focus on the safety of medicines in children. Be alert and *always* report suspected adverse reactions. Never underestimate your role in this. Reports should be filled out on the usual yellow card system and sent to the CSM. The CSM has a subgroup that specifically focuses on paediatric medicines.

4 Prescribing in Older Patients

Anthony Grosso

Older patients, especially if debilitated, deserve special thought when prescribing. We have to be careful about quantifying age with respect to 'older people' – however, ≥75 years is a good working definition.

Pharmacokinetic changes

Renal clearance capacity falls with age, meaning that older patients will eliminate some drugs and their metabolites more slowly than younger patients. Therefore, doses of some drugs (eg, digoxin) should be reduced.

Clearance can also be reduced by acute illness or dehydration – especially in older patients – so that adverse or toxic effects suddenly appear in a patient on a previously stable (and safe) dose. Indeed, older patients are often more sensitive to adverse effects, and some drugs are best avoided altogether. Meanwhile, the absorption, distribution and metabolism of some drugs is altered in older patients. You *must* therefore consult a reference source (such as the *BNF* or your pharmacist) if in any doubt.

Polypharmacy

Older patients often have multiple diseases and need multiple drugs. This increases the risk of drug–drug and drug–food interactions and the development of adverse drug reactions. Polypharmacy can also affect compliance and increase the risk of errors.

Risk–benefit

Older patients should not be denied treatment due to their age – but *do* consider the risk–benefit analysis. Warfarin might reduce stroke rates in atrial fibrillation, but is your patient unsteady on their feet?

Concordance

Can the patient handle very small tablets? Open the bottles? See the labels? Or see differences in tablet colour? Swallow big tablets? *Think!* The solution might be simple.

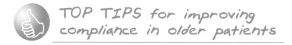

TOP TIPS for improving compliance in older patients

Review every chart every day!

- What can you cross off?

- What alternative formulations are available? Try to simplify the regimen (eg, from 6-hourly to OD administration) or employ approved combinations (eg, change amiloride 5 mg and furosemide 40 mg to co-amilofruse 5/40).

On discharge, ask yourself:

- Does the patient *really* need to be discharged taking all of those drugs?

- Have you used large-print labels for patients with visual impairment?

- Are the containers non-child-resistant for patients with arthritis?

- If the patient has a complicated drug regimen, have you given him/her a reminder chart or compliance box?

- Have you thought about the use of liquids for patients with swallowing difficulties?

- Does the patient need any help? Should a district nurse visit to administer insulin?

Prescribing in Renal Disease

Dipty Joshi

Don't *cause* renal failure!

The kidneys are desperately sensitive to damage by drugs: fully 20% of ARF episodes are drug induced! Be afraid. Be *very* afraid. And then take care:

- Identify patients at risk and, if possible, eliminate their risk factors.

- Avoid potentially nephrotoxic agents wherever possible.

- Adjust drug doses, where necessary, in all those with pre-existing renal impairment – drug accumulation and toxicity can quickly develop.

Many drugs are potentially nephrotoxic and the list is too long to remember. However, high-risk classes to *AVOID* are as follows…

ACE inhibitors and ARBs
ACE inhibitors and ARBs lower glomerular filtration pressure and can help the tubular uptake of other nephrotoxic drugs. Take care when prescribing these drugs in patients who have pre-existing renal disease, dehydration or possible renal artery stenosis, and in those who are taking other potentially nephrotoxic drugs. If you're worried, carefully monitor the patient's BP and biochemical markers of renal function.

IV contrast media/dye

Risk is particularly high in patients with pre-existing renal impairment or dehydration. In 50% of diabetics with impaired renal function, renal function declines further after the use of radiocontrast agents.

Hydration with a balanced salt solution (Hartmann's/Ringer's lactate) is a key preventative strategy. Acetylcysteine (600 mg PO BD 24 hours before and 24 hours after contrast) or a prophylactic infusion of 1.26% sodium bicarbonate can also help.

AntibiOtics

Antibiotics can be directly tubulotoxic or cause allergic interstitial nephritis or crystallisation within the renal tubules.

Aminoglycosides are a common culprit: even with proper dose adjustment there is no guarantee of safety, and nephrotoxicity still occurs at therapeutic levels. Penicillin, cephalosporin and quinolones are other offenders.

LIthium

Careful monitoring of lithium levels is *crucial*.

NSAIDs and COX-2 inhibitors

The risk rises with the dose given. If you're worried, think of alternatives.

Doubling the damage

You should especially *AVOID* using such classes in combination: gentamicin and cephalosporin in the infected renal stone patient are bad enough, but add diclofenac for the pain and…!

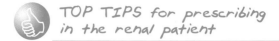

TOP TIPS for prescribing in the renal patient

To avoid drug toxicity, think of the following five points:

- Don't exceed the recommended dose.

- For patients at risk of ARF, reduce the dose, concentration and/or rate of administration.

- Where necessary, monitor drug levels closely (eg, vancomycin, gentamicin).

- Tailor the drug therapy to the individual needs of each patient with renal insufficiency. Some patients might have some residual function, which you will want to preserve for as long as possible.

- Periodic monitoring of renal function tests and urine output is particularly important in patients with renal impairment or who are at risk of developing ARF.

If in doubt, *ask your hospital pharmacist*!

Treatment of the patient with known chronic renal impairment

Ok, so now the patient has presented with chronic renal failure. What drugs might they need? Here is a rough guide!

- Hypertension – a slight decrease in BP can have a significant effect in rescuing the patient's renal function. For example, ACE inhibitors can reduce the rate of loss of function, even if the BP is normal but urea is high.

- Oedema – treatment with high doses of loop diuretics (eg, furosemide 250 mg to 2 g/day ± metolazone 5–10 mg/day) might be required.

- Renal bone disease – give phosphate binders (eg, Calcichew®) and vitamin D analogues (eg, alfacalcidol) and treat as soon as there is an increase in parathyroid hormone.

- Dietary advice – aim to restrict sodium intake as this will help to control the BP and prevent oedema. Restrict potassium if there is evidence of hyperkalaemia and acidosis, in which case treat with bicarbonate supplements. Reduce dietary phosphate intake.

- Anaemia – treat with erythropoietin. Give iron if deficient.

- Hyperlipidaemia – this will increase the risk of cardiovascular disease and contribute to renal insufficiency. Use statins as first-line.

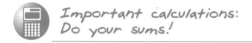

Important calculations: Do your sums!

Drug doses can be adjusted according to the patient's creatinine clearance. The most accurate method of determining creatinine clearance is to gather urine over 24 hours, and then use the following equation:

$$CrCl = UV / Pt$$

where:

CrCl = creatinine clearance

U = urinary creatinine concentration (μmol/L)

V = volume of urine (mL)

P = plasma creatinine concentration (μmol/L)

t = time (minutes)

Table 2. Definitions of renal impairment.

Grade	GFR (mL/minutes)	Serum creatinine (μmol/L)
Mild	20–50	150–300
Moderate	10–20	300–700
Severe	<10	>700

A quicker and less cumbersome method is to use the Cockcroft–Gault equation. This is widely used to measure an adult's plasma creatinine concentration and hence his/her renal function:

$$\mathrm{CrCl} = \frac{G \times (140 - \text{age in years}) \times \text{weight in kg}}{\text{serum creatinine } (\mu\mathrm{mol/L})}$$

where:

G = 1.04 (females) or 1.23 (males)

Which equation to use?

The Cockcroft–Gault equation provides an approximation of creatinine clearance, so is particularly useful when renal dysfunction is stable. It is less appropriate in a dynamic clinical setting such as ARF, where renal function can change on a daily basis and creatinine concentrations might not have reached steady state. Height and body weight are critically important to calculate drug dosages in all patients – particularly in obese or oedematous patients, use ideal body weight.

Choosing a dose

Before choosing an appropriate drug and dosage schedule, the severity of renal impairment must be assessed. This is done by estimating the GFR.

For prescribing purposes, renal impairment is divided into three broad groups (see **Table 2**): mild, moderate and severe. Armed with this classification, you are now in a position to choose the right dose from **Table 3**.

Table 3. Dosage selection in relation to the severity of renal dysfunction.
[a]Increase dose by 50% in severe infection.

Drug	CrCl (mL/minutes)	Dose
Aciclovir PO	20–50	Dose as per normal renal function
	10–20	Simplex: 200 mg TDS/QDS
		Zoster: 400–800 mg TDS
	<10	Simplex: 200 mg BD
		Zoster: 400–800 mg BD
Aciclovir IV	25–50	5–10 mg/kg BD
	10–25	5–10 mg/kg BD
	<10	2.5–5 mg/kg BD
Allopurinol	20–50	200–300 mg OD
	10–20	100–200 mg OD
	<10	100 mg OD or alternate day
Amikacin IV	20–50	5–6 mg/kg BD
	10–20	3–4 mg/kg BD
	<10	2 mg/kg every 24–48 hours
Amoxicillin PO/IV	20–50	Dose as per normal renal function
	10–20	Dose as per normal renal function
	<10	250 mg TDS
Amphotericin IV	<50	Seek advice
Azathioprine	20–50	Dose as per normal renal function
	10–20	75–100% of normal dose
	<10	50–75% of normal dose
Benzylpenicillin IV	20–50	Dose as per normal renal function
	10–20	75% of normal dose
	<10	20–50% of normal dose
Bisoprolol	20–50	Dose as per normal renal function
	10–20	Dose as per normal renal function
	<10	1.25–10 mg OD
Cefotaxime IV	20–50	Dose as per normal renal function
	10–20	Dose as per normal renal function
	<10	Load with 1 g then half daily dose at same frequency

Table 3. *Continued.*

Drug	CrCl (mL/minutes)	Dose
Ceftazidime IV	30–50	1 g BD[a]
	15–30	1 g OD[a]
	5–15	500 mg to 1 g OD[a]
	<5	500 mg to 1 g 48-hourly[a]
Ceftriaxone IV	20–50	Dose as per normal renal function
	<10	Dose as per normal renal function
		Use with caution in patients with severe renal impairment as well as in patients with hepatic insufficiency
		In severe infection, dose at 1 g OD and increase to 2 g if necessary
Cefuroxime IV	20–50	750 mg to 1.5 g TDS
	10–20	750 mg to 1.5 g BD/TDS
	<10	1.5 g OD
Chloral hydrate	20–50	Dose as per normal renal function
	10–20	500 mg nocte
	<10	Avoid
Ciprofloxacin	20–50	Dose as per normal renal function
	10–20	50% of normal dose
	<10	50% of normal dose
Clarithromycin PO	20–50	Dose as per normal renal function
	10–20	250–500 mg OD/BD
	<10	250 mg OD/BD
Clarithromycin IV	20–50	Dose as per normal renal function
	10–20	250–500 mg BD
	<10	250 mg BD
Clindamycin	10–50	Dose as per normal renal function
Co-amoxiclav PO	30–50	Dose as per normal renal function
	10–30	Dose as per normal renal function
	<10	375 mg TDS
Co-amoxiclav IV	30–50	Dose as per normal renal function
	10–30	1.2 g BD
	<10	1.2 g stat followed by 600 mg to 1.2 g OD

Table 3. *Continued.*

Drug	CrCl (mL/minutes)	Dose
Co-codamol/ co-dydramol	20–50	Dose as per normal renal function
	10–20	75–100% of normal dose
Co-trimoxazole PO/IV	>25	Dose as per normal renal function
	15–25	Normal dose for 3 days then half standard dose
	<15	To be given if haemodialysis facilities are available
		Normal dose for 3 days then half standard dose
Doxazosin	–	Dose as per normal renal function
Doxycycline	–	Dose as per normal renal function
Enalapril	20–50	Dose as per normal renal function
	10–20	Start with 2.5 mg/day then dose to response
	<10	Start with 2.5 mg/day then dose to response
Erythromycin	20–50	Dose as per normal renal function
	10–20	Dose as per normal renal function
	<10	50–75% of normal dose, maximum 1.5 g/day
Ethambutol	20–50	Dose as per normal renal function
	10–20	Normal dose 24- to 36-hourly
	<10	Normal dose 48-hourly
Flucloxacillin	20–50	Dose as per normal renal function
	<10–20	Dose as per normal renal function
Fluconazole	20–50	Dose as per normal renal function
	10–20	Dose as per normal renal function
	<10	50% of normal dose
Foscarnet IV	<50	See local guidelines
Gabapentin	60–90	400 mg TDS
	30–60	300 mg BD
	15–30	300 mg OD
	<15	300 mg 48-hourly

Table 3. *Continued.*

Drug	CrCl (mL/minutes)	Dose
Ganciclovir IV	>70	5 mg/kg BD
	50–70	2.5 mg/kg BD
	25–50	2.5 mg/kg OD
	10–25	1.25 mg/kg OD
	<10	1.25 mg/kg OD
Gentamicin	<50	See local guidelines
Haloperidol	20–50	Dose as per normal renal function
	10–20	Dose as per normal renal function
	<10	Start with lower dose; will accumulate
Heparin	<50	Dose as per normal renal function
Hydroxyurea	20–50	100% of normal dose
	10–20	50% of normal dose and titrate to response
	<10	20% of normal dose and titrate to response
Imipenem	30–50	500 mg TDS/QDS
	20–30	500 mg BD/TDS
	10–20	250–500 mg BD
	<10	250 mg BD
Isosorbide di/mononitrate	<50	Dose as per normal renal function
Itraconazole	<50	Dose as per normal renal function
Labetalol	<50	Dose as per normal renal function
Lansoprazole	<50	Dose as per normal renal function
Levothyroxine	<50	Dose as per normal renal function
Linezolid PO/IV	<50	Dose as per normal renal function
Meropenem	20–50	500 mg to 1 g BD
	10–20	250 mg to 1 g BD or 500 mg TDS
	<10	250 mg to 1 g OD
Metformin	40–50	25–50% of dose
	10–40	Avoid
	<10	Avoid

Table 3. *Continued.*

Drug	CrCl (mL/minutes)	Dose
Methyldopa	20–50	250–500 mg TDS
	10–20	250–500 mg BD/TDS
	<10	250–500 mg OD/BD
Morphine	20–50	75% of normal dose
	10–20	Use small doses, eg, 2.5–5 mg
	<10	Use small doses, eg, 1.25–2.5 mg
Oxytetracycline	20–50	Dose as per normal renal function
	10–20	500 mg to 1 g OD
	<10	500 mg to 1 g 48-hourly
Penicillin V	<50	Dose as per normal renal function
Phenytoin	<50	Dose as per normal renal function
Pyrazinamide	10–50	Dose as per normal renal function
	<10	Reduce size or frequency of dose
Rifampicin	10–50	Dose as per normal renal function
	<10	50–100% of normal dose
Sodium fusidate	–	Dose as per normal renal function
Sodium valproate	<50	Dose as per normal renal function
Sotalol	20–50	50% of normal dose
	10–20	25% of normal dose
	<10	Avoid
Streptomycin	<50	Reduce dose and measure levels
Tamoxifen	<50	Dose as per normal renal function
Tazocin	20–50	Dose as per normal renal function
	10–20	4.5 g BD
	<10	4.5 g BD
Teicoplanin		Normal dose for first 3 days then reduce
	40–50	Give standard dose on alternate days
	<40	Give standard dose every third day
Tramadol	20–50	Dose as per normal renal function
	10–20	50–100 mg BD
	<10	50 mg BD

Table 3. *Continued.*

Drug	CrCl (mL/minutes)	Dose
Trimethoprim	>25	Dose as per normal renal function
	15–25	Normal dose for 3 days then half normal dose 18-hourly
	<10	Half normal dose OD
Urokinase	<50	Dose as per normal renal function
Valaciclovir	30–50	Dose as per normal renal function
	15–30	Herpes simplex: Dose as per normal renal function
		Herpes zoster: 1 g OD/BD
	<15	Herpes simplex: 500 mg OD
		Herpes zoster: 500 mg to 1 g OD
Valganciclovir	40–60	Induction/treatment: 450 mg BD
		Maintenance/prophylaxis: 450 mg OD
	25–40	Induction/treatment: 450 mg OD
		Maintenance/prophylaxis: 450 mg 48-hourly
	10–25	Induction/treatment: 450 mg 48-hourly
		Maintenance/prophylaxis: 450 mg twice weekly
	<10	Treatment: 450 mg twice weekly
Vancomycin	20–50	1 g stat and adjust according to levels
	<20	1 g stat and monitor serum levels at 24-hour intervals
Venlafaxine	30–50	Dose as per normal renal function
	10–30	Reduce dose by 50% and administer OD
	<10	Reduce dose by 50% and administer OD
Warfarin	<50	Dose as per normal renal function
Zopiclone	10–50	Dose as per normal renal function
	<10	50–100% of normal dose

6 Treating Diabetes

Preet Panesar

Intravenous insulin infusions

In diabetics, it can be hard to control glucose levels during illness and peri-operatively – glucose levels are affected by counter-regulatory hormones, unpredictable eating (eg, illness, NBM, changing meal times), changing IV glucose rates, lack of exercise, unusual timing of insulin injections and medications (eg, glucocorticoids, catecholamines). Despite these difficulties, tight control is particularly important: it improves outcome in critically ill hospitalised patients and reduces infection rates.

A variety of different methods have emerged to administer continuous IV insulin. A few examples of the different regimens are given below. *Find out the local guidelines at your hospital and use those.*

Regimens

Sliding-scale

- Insulin is given via a syringe driver: 50 units soluble insulin in 50 mL sodium chloride 0.9% (ie, 1 unit/mL). This is connected via a three-way tap to a bag of dextrose (eg, glucose 10% with 20 mmol potassium).

- The dextrose is infused at a constant rate (eg, 80 mL/hour).

- The insulin infusion is started at 2–4 units/hour. If the patient has previously been on insulin then you should divide the patient's usual total daily dose of insulin by 24 and start at this rate (eg, 48 units in 24 hours – start at 2 units/hour).

Table 4. Sliding-scale insulin infusion regimens.

Blood glucose level (mmol/L)	Insulin infusion rate (units/hour)		
	Regimen 1	Regimen 2	Regimen 3
<4	0.5	1	2
4–10	2	4	8
10–15	4	8	16
15–20	6	12	24
>20	Review	Review	Review

- The insulin infusion rate is changed according to a predefined scale that is solely dependent on blood glucose levels (as shown in regimen 1, **Table 4**).

- Blood glucose levels are initially monitored hourly until stable, then 4-hourly.

- Some hospitals have two or three different regimens. Patients will start on regimen 1. Those who are resistant to insulin or who still have uncontrolled blood glucose levels will be moved onto regimen 2 and then, if still uncontrolled, onto regimen 3 (see **Table 4**).

The sliding scale has been criticised for 'chasing' blood glucose levels, leading to erratic increases and decreases in blood glucose.

Dose titration

As opposed to the sliding-scale regimen, the dose-titration regimen prompts a change in the insulin infusion rate only once a *trend* towards increasing or decreasing blood glucose levels has been seen.

- Set up an insulin infusion with a bag of glucose, as for the sliding-scale regimen.

- Define the blood glucose range for nursing staff (eg, "Keep blood glucose levels within 6–10 mmol/L").

- Nursing staff then adjust insulin infusion rates on their own initiative, according to the trend in blood glucose levels.

Example

- Prescription: 50 units Actrapid® in 50 mL NaCl 0.9%. Start at 2 units/hour. Keep blood glucose within 6–10 mmol/L.

- Check blood glucose levels hourly.

- If blood glucose is *increasing* on two consecutive readings, *increase* the insulin infusion rate by 0.5–2 units/hour.

- If blood glucose is *decreasing* on two consecutive readings, *decrease* the insulin infusion rate by 0.5–2 units/hour.

- If the blood glucose is ≤3 mmol/L, *stop* the insulin infusion and treat as for hypoglycaemia (see **Section 2, Chapter 3**). Restart the infusion after reducing the original infusion rate by 1–2 units/hour.

Glucose–potassium–insulin infusion

A further alternative is the glucose–potassium–insulin regimen (GKI, GIK or Alberti regimen). This was introduced as a novel method of improving glycaemic control in the peri-operative period. Variations of this regimen are used in MI patients, where it confers prognostic benefit.

- Glucose, potassium and insulin, in the same container, are infused at a constant rate.

- Blood glucose levels are monitored hourly.

- The rate of infusion remains constant, but the amount of insulin in the bag is changed depending on the blood glucose levels.

Example

- Set up an infusion of dextrose 10% with 20 mmol/L potassium and 15 units of soluble insulin. Run it at a rate appropriate to the patient's fluid requirements, usually 80 mL/hour. (Obese patients or those on large amounts`of insulin will need more insulin added to the bag.)

- Check the patient's blood glucose levels 1- to 2-hourly. Aim to keep the blood glucose between 6 and 10 mmol/L.

- If the blood glucose is >10 mmol/L and rising (ie, two consecutive values show an increase) or steady, take down the infusion bag and replace it with one containing an additional 4 units of soluble insulin. Run the new bag at the same rate of 80 mL/hour and reassess after 1–2 hours.

- If the blood glucose is 6–10 mmol/L, maintain the current regimen and infusion rate.

- If the blood glucose is <6 mmol/L and falling (ie, two consecutive values show a decrease), take down the infusion bag and replace it with one containing 4 units less of soluble insulin than previously. Run the new bag at the same rate of 80 mL/hour, and reassess after 1–2 hours.

- If the blood glucose is ≤3mmol/L, *stop* the infusion and take down the infusion bag. Treat the patient for hypoglycaemia (see **Section 2, Chapter 3**). Prepare a new bag with 4 units less of insulin, and restart the infusion at 80 mL/hour.

The bags should also be changed if potassium requirements increase or decrease.

Table 5. Pharmacokinetic profiles of various insulin preparations.

Insulin type	Onset	Peak	Duration
Rapid acting:			
Humalog® (insulin lispro)	Within 15 minutes	30 minutes to 1 hour	2–5 hours
NovoRapid® (insulin aspart)			
Short acting:			
Human Actrapid®	30 minutes	1–3 hours	6–8 hours
Humulin S®			
Intermediate acting:			
Human Insulatard®	2 hours	4–12 hours	Up to 24 hours (considerable patient variation)
Humulin I®			
Long-acting analogues:			
Lantus® (insulin glargine)	1 hour	Flat	24 hours
Detemir® (insulin levemir)			
Mixed insulins (biphasic):			
NovoMix 30®	Up to 2 hours	4–12 hours	Up to 24 hours
Humalog Mix® 25, 50			
Human Mixtard® 10, 20, 30, 40, 50			
Humulin M3®			

Insulin preparations

Table 5 will familiarise you with the more common insulin preparations. Preparations differ in their pharmacokinetics. Note that action profiles can be affected by the dose, injection site and technique, exercise and temperature.

Table 6. Oral hypoglycaemic agents. [a]See *BNF* for the complete list.

Agent	Indications	Action	Side effects[a]	Contraindications	Timing	Example
Biguanides	Obese, first or second line	↑ insulin sensitivity	Nausea, abdominal pain, diarrhoea	Liver, renal or heart failure Care with contrast media Pregnancy	Take on a full stomach	Metformin
Sulphonylureas	Non-obese, first or second line Unable to tolerate metformin	↑ insulin secretion	Weight gain, hypoglycaemia	Severe liver or renal failure Pregnancy Avoid long-acting preparations in the elderly	15–30 minutes before food	Gliclazide, glibenclamide, glipizide, glimepiride, tolbutamide
Alpha-glucosidase inhibitors	Obese, second or third line	↓ intestinal absorption	Abdominal pain, flatus, diarrhoea	Severe liver or renal failure Pregnancy Inflammatory bowel disease or obstruction	Just before food or with first mouthful of food	Acarbose
Thiazolidinediones (glitazones)	Second line (as per NICE guidance) In combination either with metformin or a sulphonylurea	↓ insulin resistance	Weight gain, oedema, liver impairment, increased LDL-cholesterol (only with rosiglitazone)	Liver impairment Heart failure Pregnancy Not licensed for use with insulin	Just before food	Pioglitazone, rosiglitazone
Prandial glucose regulators	Non-obese, second or third line Unable to tolerate metformin	↑ insulin release	Hypoglycaemia, weight gain, abdominal pain, diarrhoea	Ketoacidosis Severe liver impairment Pregnancy	Within 30 minutes before food	Repaglinide, nateglinide

Oral hypoglycaemic agents

The choice of oral hypoglycaemic agents is shown in **Table 6**. Commencing a patient newly diagnosed with diabetes on medication is difficult: *seek specialist advice!*

7

Management of the Acutely Confused Patient

Hugh Montgomery

Acute confusion can present with paranoia (bombs under the bed; you are an enemy agent), aggression or more subtly (the patient is packed and asking for a cab home at 3 am). Ultimately, treatment should be directed at the cause.

- Sometimes, it is *simple disorientation.* Most of what we do in hospital (a strange environment, disrupted day/night cycle, odd drugs, random awakenings, sleep deprivation/disruption, noise, pain) is used to 'break' prisoners in wartime and is banned by the Geneva Convention. Try to prevent such factors! Older patients are much more vulnerable.

- *Drug or alcohol withdrawal* are also common causes. See the next chapter for the prevention of DTs.

- *Organic medical causes.* Think especially of metabolic causes, eg, hypo- or hyperglycaemia/disrupted sodium or water balance/acidosis; hypoperfusion (low cardiac output); infection (note: there may be no other signs, especially in older patients); respiratory failure (low O_2 or high CO_2).

Now, here is the problem. You are always told that: "It's dangerous to sedate a patient when there could be an organic cause" – but the patient won't let you near them to examine them/send blood tests/get an X-ray. You sit there for hours trying to be reasonable and get nowhere. So what do you do?

Restraint and environment

You might *have* to sedate the patient in order to be able to investigate and treat them – for their own good and safety.

- This might need restraint from suitably trained staff (eg, security/other medical or nursing staff) to allow you to administer a sedative. *This is important!* Overzealous behaviour – such as leaning on the 20-stone man who is fighting hard – can compress the chest enough to kill the patient.

- In any case, make sure that the environment is safe: that the patient or staff won't be injured by a fall, for instance. Do you want a mattress on the floor? Or cot-sides up afterwards?

- If you use IV sedatives, have monitoring facilities to hand, and ideally an available bed on a suitable ward (such as the HDU).

Dose and route of administration of sedative

Give small, repeat doses. Once they're in, large doses can't be taken back out. If given IM, you might be unaware of the overdose until hours later.

- Give a tablet if you can. (However, in this state, few patients will agree!)

- If no venous access is available, use the IM route.

- If venous access is available (or can be obtained without injury to the patient) then put a safe maximum in the syringe (with a mobile patient, accidental emptying of the syringe can happen) having diluted the drug, and then give a small bolus, then another, then another – and wait until you have the effect that you want *and no more*. If you need a sustained effect, a small IM dose of another agent can be used a while later.

The drugs of choice

Here are your options:

- Chlorpromazine (25–100 mg PO/IM) has more sedative effects than haloperidol (5–10 mg PO or 5–7.5 mg IM). Both can cause hypotension and respiratory depression in excessive dosage. Where possible, wait 20 minutes before administering a further dose. *Procyclidine should be available PO/IM to treat extrapyramidal side effects.*

- Use benzodiazepines if there is a history of cardiac disease. Lorazepam (2–4 mg PO or up to 50 μg/kg IV/IM) is useful and has lower tissue accumulation than diazepam (2.5–10 mg PO/IM). Flumazenil should be available if respiratory depression occurs. Administer, and call the ICU (as the reversal will wear off!).

 TOP TIPS in sedation

Important points to note are:

- Use half of these doses in older patients.

- Always correct and prevent hypoxaemia: all sedated patients should receive oxygen.

- Sometimes the hypoxic patient needs sedation in order to keep the mask on! If this is the case, *don't do the sedating* – the patient should probably be in an HDU facility.

Alcohol Dependence and the DTs

8

Rob Shulman

Do not take alcohol withdrawal lightly. It can be lethal through its physiological consequences, direct injury (jumping from a window) or non-compliance (pulling out chest drains or drips). Find out what local facilities are available for the longer-term management of alcoholics. The following guidelines are for in-patients only.

In dealing with alcohol dependence and withdrawal, there are two headlines:

Headline 1: think of drink!

Always, ALWAYS, *ALWAYS* ask about alcohol consumption – and make it clear that you are non-judgemental. Remember to be suspicious: assume that most people (just like you!) underestimate their consumption.

Look for clues that there might be an alcohol problem. Is the MCV high? Are there healed fractures on the chest X-ray? Is the patient's history compatible with excess intake?

Headline 2: a preventative measure

A heavy drinker, deprived of alcohol for a day or two, will get the DTs. Guaranteed. This usually happens between days 2 and 5, but can come on earlier (eg, ≤24 hours). You have five choices when dealing with the dependent:

1. Discuss the issue and allow them to drink responsibly while in hospital, if this fits with the pattern of investigation and treatment.

2. Prescribe a steady background of medication to stop them withdrawing from alcohol.

3. Prescribe a reducing dose of medication so that they can safely withdraw (if they want to stop drinking).

4. Watch like a hawk for worrying signs (eg, rising pulse rate, tremor, sweatiness, agitation) and *act smartly to treat,* or…

5. …be a total idiot. Ignore the issue. Face the consequences.

Drug management of DTs

Remember, one size doesn't fit all. Sedative doses should be tailored to the individual's requirements. This requires review at least once daily.

Preventing DTs and managing them after mild onset

There are a variety of regimens available for this purpose. However, chlordiazepoxide is the drug of choice. Initially, 30 mg QDS should be adequate, but in severe cases you can increase the dose to a maximum of 50 mg QDS. For nighttime sedation, give a larger dose (eg, double the daytime dose) at bedtime and the ward will enjoy a quieter night! Take care when prescribing for a patient who is intoxicated or sedated.

If you opt for controlled withdrawal, **Table 7** gives a suggested oral reducing regimen (titrate according to the patient's response). Prescribe 20 mg PRN on top of this. Doses can be reduced if necessary (eg, in older patients).

Table 7. Chlordiazepoxide dosing regimen for the prevention of DTs.

Day	Time			
	0800	1200	1800	2200
	Chlordiazepoxide dose (mg)			
1	30	30	30	30
2	25	25	25	25
3	20	20	20	20
4	10	10	10	20
5	5	5	5	10
6	–	5	5	10
7	–	–	5	5
8	–	–	–	5

Alternatives to chlordiazepoxide

- Lorazepam has a shorter duration of action than chlordiazepoxide and might be preferable in older patients or in those with severe hepatic dysfunction (0.5 mg lorazepam ~ 15 mg chlordiazepoxide).

- Diazepam should be used if the parenteral or rectal routes are required (5 mg diazepam ~ 15 mg chlordiazepoxide).

- Clomethiazole (chlormethiazole) is useful if the patient is sensitive to benzodiazepines, but beware the increased risk of respiratory depression if the patient goes on an alcohol bender. A good option is to use Heminevrin® capsules (192 mg chlormethiazole):

  – 3 capsules QDS on day 1
  – 3 capsules TDS on day 2
  – 2 capsules TDS on day 3
  – 1 capsule QDS on day 4
  – 1 capsule TDS on day 5

Don't give the patient any chlormethiazole to take home.

Whichever drug and regimen you use, think of a larger dose last thing at night, reduce doses if sleepy and increase if signs of DTs are escalating.

Adjuncts to chlordiazepoxide

Continue any established anti-epileptic drugs. For patients who are not on any anti-convulsant but who are known to be susceptible to seizures, prescribe carbamazepine 200 mg PO 12-hourly during detoxification. Use diazepam 10 mg IV/PR stat if chlordiazepoxide does not adequately control seizures. Consider propranolol 40 mg PO 8- to 12-hourly (or higher) PRN for reducing sweating, palpitations and tremor if the patient is particularly distressed.

Treating acute severe DTs

See the previous chapter.

Prevention of Wernicke–Korsakoff syndrome

Remember: This condition can cause permanent disability. *Prevent it!*

On admission, administer parenteral Pabrinex® to all alcohol-dependent patients who are due to undergo in-patient alcohol withdrawal, or to those patients who are thought to be severely thiamine deficient. Pabrinex contains vitamins B and C, but you are using it for the thiamine content. Pabrinex should be administered before any parenteral glucose is given.

Prevention of Wernicke's encephalopathy

One pair of Pabrinex IVHP ampoules OD/BD for 3–5 days.

Therapeutic treatment for Wernicke's encephalopathy

Two pairs of Pabrinex IVHP ampoules TDS for 3 days, then review. If no response is seen, discontinue therapy; if a response is seen, decrease the dose to *one* pair of ampoules daily, given for as long as improvement continues.

When the Pabrinex course is finished, give oral thiamine 50 mg TDS and 1–2 multivitamin tablets daily, usually for the rest of the admission. For severe vitamin B group deficiency, give 1–2 vitamin B compound strong tablets TDS. A short course of folic acid 5 mg PO OD might also be beneficial.

2

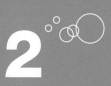

Emergency Prescribing

1. Diabetic Ketoacidosis   51
2. Hyperosmolar Non-ketotic Coma   53
3. Hypoglycaemia   55
4. Paracetamol Overdose   57
5. Emergency Prescribing in Cardiology   60
6. Emergency Prescribing in Neurosurgery   68
7. Massive Pulmonary Embolism   73
8. Electrolyte and Metabolic Emergencies   75
9. Respiratory Emergencies   82

Diabetic Ketoacidosis

Preet Panesar

DKA is a life-threatening triad of hyperglycaemia, ketonuria and acidosis. It is more common in uncontrolled type 1 diabetes, but can also occur in type 2 diabetes in response to acute stress. Some useful tips in prescribing include...

Insulin

Prescribe soluble insulin (human Actrapid®), given via a syringe, at a concentration of 1 unit/mL – give a stat dose of 6 units IV, then infuse at a rate of 6 units/hour (or 0.1 units/kg/hour for children). Check blood glucose levels hourly and aim to reduce blood glucose by 2–4 mmol/L/hour.

Fluids

Correct fluids over 24–48 hours.

- You will probably need to replace 6 L (or 100 mL/kg) of fluid. Typically, replace 1 L/hour for the first 2 hours, then reduce the rate of infusion. The infusion rate should be modified according to age, cardiac history, shock, hypotension, degree of dehydration and urinary output.

- Once blood glucose falls below 15 mmol/L, replace with 10% glucose.

Potassium

Avoid potassium replacement with the first litre of fluid or if the potassium level is >5.5 mmol/L.

- About 200–300 mmol of potassium will need to be replaced over 24–48 hours.

- Check the potassium level every 2 hours for the first 6 hours, then every 6 hours thereafter.

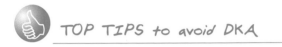

TOP TIPS to avoid DKA

Some post-episode counselling for patients will stop them coming into hospital again! Give them this advice for periods of illness:

- Even if you are not eating, *never ever* stop insulin. You *must* continue to take your normal dose.

- Test your blood at least four times a day, and test your urine for ketones at least twice a day.

- If your glucose and ketone levels are high, you might need to increase your insulin dose. Check with your diabetic team.

- If you can't eat solid foods, try to replace them with alternatives such as Lucozade or other sugary drinks, soup, milk, ice-cream, honey, boiled sweets or glucose tablets.

Hyperosmolar Non-ketotic Coma

2

Preet Panesar

Hyperosmolar non-ketotic coma is usually seen in uncontrolled type 2 diabetes mellitus. As the name suggests, these patients tend to have very high blood glucose levels without any acidosis, and they are also severely dehydrated. The majority of cases occur in middle-aged or elderly patients. Two thirds of cases occur in previously undiagnosed patients.

The principles of treatment are similar to those of DKA, but there are some subtle differences. Some useful tips in prescribing include:

Fluids

* Give 0.9% sodium chloride IV.

* You will probably need to replace between 5 and 9 L of fluid. The infusion rate should be adjusted according to age, cardiac history, dehydration and urinary output. Watch the fluid balance carefully.

* Once blood glucose falls below 15 mmol/L, replace with 10% glucose.

Potassium

* Only start when renal function is satisfactory or the plasma potassium level is low.

* Requirements are less than for DKA – around 100 mmol of potassium will need to be replaced over 24–48 hours.

Insulin

- Start the infusion at 3–4 units/hour and titrate
  to maintain a blood glucose of 4–8 mmol/L.

Hypoglycaemia

3

Preet Panesar

Left untreated, hypoglycaemia can cause accidents, fits, permanent brain injury or even death. Symptoms tend to occur when blood glucose falls below 3 mmol/L (although this varies). The patient might be unaware of the symptoms – sleepiness (coma being mistaken for sleep), altered personality (eg, aggression), poor concentration, sweating or confusion can also be easily missed by hospital staff.

A variety of triggers make attacks more likely in hospitals. Irregular eating habits, delaying meals, NBM, inability to absorb food and recent changes in medication and doses all put the patient at risk.

Episodes can be divided into mild–moderate and severe. The treatment depends on which category the patient falls into.

Mild–moderate hypoglycaemia

- The patient should be given 10–15 g of carbohydrate (eg, 2 cubes or a teaspoon of sugar, 2–3 glucose tablets, 2 teaspoons of honey, 200 mL Lucozade, 90 mL cola). They should then start to feel better within 10 minutes. Follow with a long-acting carbohydrate (eg, biscuits, bread) to prevent recurrence.

- If the patient is semi-conscious, place GlucoGel® glucose gel inside his/her cheek and gently rub the outside of the cheek to allow absorption through the lining of the mouth. *Do not* give this if the patient is unconscious – it will go down the wrong way.

Severe hypoglycaemia

- Give IV glucose – 100 mL of 20% glucose or 250 mL of 10% glucose. Ideally, these should be given in a big vein as they are irritant, but not as irritant as 50% glucose! Patients usually respond quickly. Follow this with a long-acting carbohydrate meal.

- Glucagon can also be given by IV, SC or IM routes (an advantage if the patient is fitting).

 RED ALERT
when giving glucagon

- Glucagon is slower than IV glucose (it can take 10–15 minutes to see an improvement).

- It is ineffective in patients with low glycogen stores (eg, starved patients, alcoholics, the elderly, those with frequent episodes of hypoglycaemia).

- *Do not* give to type 2 diabetics! These patients have reserves of endogenous insulin – glucagon stimulates insulin release and can make the hypoglycaemia worse.

Paracetamol Overdose

4

Jane Ng
(with acknowledgement to Jonathan Robin)

Paracetamol overdose is common and can prove fatal: as little as 10–15 g (20–30 tablets) can cause severe hepatocellular failure, acute renal tubular necrosis (rarely) and then death 3–4 days later.

There are two treatment strategies:

- decrease absorption, or…

- …support the non-toxic metabolism of the drug

Decreasing absorption

Multi-dose activated charcoal (50 g stat, then every 4 hours) reduces paracetamol absorption *only* if given within 1 hour of overdose. You should routinely give anti-emetics with the charcoal, and reduce the dose and raise the frequency if it is still not tolerated (eg, 25 g 2-hourly or 12.5 g hourly). Gastric lavage can be used up to 2 hours after overdose.

Metabolic manipulation

NAC aids the metabolism of paracetamol down a non-hepatotoxin-producing pathway. Prescribe as an IV infusion in a 5% glucose solution.

- Initial dosing is 150 mg/kg in 200 mL of 5% glucose over 15 minutes.

- Then, 50 mg/kg in 500 mL over 4 hours.

- Then, 100 mg/kg in 1 L over 16 hours.

If you know when the overdose was taken

Give NAC within 10–12 hours of ingestion, if eligible: take blood >4 hours following overdose (earlier = inaccurate) to establish the paracetamol level, then refer to the nomogram in the *BNF*. Treat if levels are above the treatment 'normal' line, or if above the 'high-risk' line if the patient is in a high-risk category. *Beware!* Toxicity can develop at lower paracetamol levels in patients on enzyme-inducing drugs or who are malnourished (eg, as a result of alcoholism or HIV).

Late presentation (>8 hours after overdose)

Treat with NAC at once. Take the paracetamol level. Continue treatment based on this level and the patient's risk status.

Very late presentation (>24 hours after overdose)

Don't go it alone! Take advice from your hospital's liver unit!

If the overdose was staggered or of unknown timing

If in doubt, *treat!* Give activated charcoal and NAC, and continue for >24 hours. If NAC is unavailable, give oral methionine (2.5 g stat, then three further doses of 2.5 g every 4 hours). Then give NAC when available.

TOP TIPS when first dealing
with a paracetamol overdose

- Beware the well patient who has taken a paracetamol
  overdose! *Do not* discharge. Admit, monitor and treat!

- *Never* take the word of a patient who has taken an
  overdose – they might have taken a far greater dose
  than they recollect.

- *Always* screen for other drugs that they might have
  taken, too – especially salicylates.

- Refer *early* for discussion with a liver unit if INR
  or LFTs are already deranged.

- *Do not* correct an abnormal INR without having
  talked with the liver unit first! It can be the best
  guide to assess the need for transplantation.

Emergency Prescribing in Cardiology

David Brull

The key conditions requiring 'cardiological emergency prescribing' are ACS, acute pulmonary oedema and acute dysrhythmia. All are scary – the patient's chest pain, hyperventilation and palpitations often seem contagious, being felt by the nurses and doctors too!

Acute coronary syndromes

ACS represent partial or complete clot occlusion of a coronary artery. They present in diverse ways – as anginal chest pain at rest or on mild exertion, with or without either ECG changes or a rise in cardiac enzymes. For all:

- high-flow oxygen (eg, 10 L via a face mask)

- analgesia with an anti-emetic:

  – diamorphine 2.5–5 mg IV/SC PRN

  – metoclopramide 10 mg PO/IV/IM TDS

- anti-platelet agents

  – aspirin 300 mg PO stat, then 75 mg PO OD

  – clopidogrel 300 mg PO stat, then (if high risk) 75 mg PO OD

  – consider a PPI, especially in older patients, to prevent stomach ulcers

- beta-blocker (BP allowing):

    – metoprolol 25 mg PO BD/TDS

    – changing to bisoprolol 2.5–10 mg PO OD once stable

    – if contraindicated, again BP allowing, consider
    slow-release verapamil or diltiazem

Diabetics need strict glycaemic control. They should have
an insulin infusion for 24 hours, followed by an insulin SC
TDS/QDS regimen for 3 months, aiming for blood sugar
levels of 4–8 mmol/L.

Non-ST-elevation MI

- LMWH – enoxaparin 1 mg/kg SC BD or dalteparin
  120 U/kg SC BD to a maximum of 10,000 U BD

- Nitrate infusion, titrating to pain and BP (maintain
  tissue perfusion and urine output).

- Risk assess all patients (eg, TIMI risk score).
  High-risk patients benefit from an early invasive
  approach involving urgent coronary angiography
  with a view to revascularisation.

ST-elevation MI

If the patient is aged <75 years, or has had previous
streptokinase, give:

- tenecteplase IV weight-adjusted bolus (500–600 µg/kg,
  maximum 50 mg) over 10 seconds, followed
  immediately by…

- …enoxaparin 1 mg/kg SC BD until discharge or …

- …unfractionated heparin, aiming for an APTT ratio
  of 1.5–2 (see **Section 5, Chapter 2**)

Consider primary PCI, where available, as the reperfusion
therapy of choice in many hospitals.

If the patient is aged >75 years, give:

- streptokinase 1.5 MU in 100 mL normal saline over 1 hour

Secondary prevention

On day 1 following an acute coronary event you should be thinking about secondary prevention:

- cholesterol-lowering therapy – statin (eg, simvastatin 40 mg PO OD, changing to atorvastatin 40 mg PO OD if total cholesterol >4 mmol/L)

- ACE inhibitor, once haemodynamically stable (eg, ramipril 5 mg PO BD)

- if the patient has a cough – losartan up to 50 mg PO BD

- antihypertensive treatment – aiming for BP <140/80 mm Hg

- smoking cessation

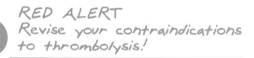

RED ALERT
Revise your contraindications to thrombolysis!

Contraindications include:

- active bleeding or bleeding disorder

- stroke/transient ischaemic attack/major surgery/ significant trauma within 2 months

- childbirth/trauma/prolonged CPR within 2 weeks

- hypertension (BP >180/110 mm Hg) – treat with nitrates/beta-blockers and reconsider thrombolysis

Note that:

- Hypotension/hypertension can be a manifestation of inadequate pain control.

- Shock is not a contraindication (and referral for percutaneous coronary intervention consideration is mandatory).

- Warfarin therapy is not a contraindication if INR is in the therapeutic range.

Acute severe pulmonary oedema

For all:

- high-flow oxygen (monitor oxygen saturations and arterial blood gases)

- opioid with anti-emetic:

  – diamorphine 2.5–5 mg IV/SC PRN

  – metoclopramide 10 mg PO/IV/IM TDS

- nitrate infusion titrating to BP, 50 mg in 50 mL of normal saline run at 2 mL/hour, titrate to pain and systolic BP >90–100 mm Hg

- consider furosemide (particularly if fluid overloaded), 40–80 mg IV stat

- discuss with ICU early!

If cardiogenic shock is present, you must discuss the patient with your tertiary cardiology referral centre – this is now mandatory!

Further specific therapy will depend on the cause or exacerbating factors of failure. Consider:

- ACS, valvular heart disease, cardiomyopathy

- infection, arrhythmia, uraemia

TOP TIPS for the management of acute severe pulmonary oedema

- Stop beta-blockers, unless failure is rate-related (eg, fast AF, high rate in hypertrophic cardiomyopathy, mitral stenosis).

- Continuous positive airway pressure or biphasic positive airway pressure can be additional therapeutic measures.

- Mechanical ventilation and inotropes might be required.

Arrhythmias

For any of the tachyarrhythmias, if the patient is haemodynamically compromised, you should consider emergency DC cardioversion. Remember to 'sync' the defibrillator. Failing that…

New-onset atrial fibrillation

AF of duration <48 hours

- Correct the electrolyte imbalance – aim for K⁺ 4.5–5 mmol/L.

- LMWH (treatment dose) – see **Section 5, Chapter 2**.

- Attempt chemical cardioversion

  – sotalol 80 mg PO BD, or…

  – …flecainide 50–100 mg BD, or…

  – …flecainide 2 mg/kg IV over 30 minutes

  – ensure continuous ECG monitoring

  – *do not* mix drugs

- Failing chemical cardioversion, and within 48 hours of symptom onset, consider DC cardioversion.

AF of duration >48 hours/unsuccessful chemical cardioversion

- Consider transoesophageal echocardiography – if there is no intracardiac thrombus, use DC cardioversion.

- If transoesophageal echocardiography is not available or if a thrombus is present:

   – anti-coagulate on warfarin (see **Section 5, Chapter 1**)

   – plan elective DC cardioversion in 4–6 weeks

Remember to consider possible causes (eg, ACS, infection, drugs, alcohol, thyrotoxicosis) and treat them if possible.

Supraventricular tachycardia

Don't panic – supraventricular tachycardias are usually well tolerated! Set up continuous ECG monitoring.

First-line therapies include vagal manoeuvres, such as carotid sinus massage, Valsalva or diving reflex.

Failing that, try adenosine (contraindicated in asthma):

- Warn the patient about chest tightness/flushing (this lasts <20 seconds).

- Using a large vein, inject a bolus of adenosine 3 mg, 6 mg, 9 mg, then 12 mg, followed by a rapid bolus of saline flush, allowing 30 seconds between increments to assess the patient's response.

- Adenosine will terminate the tachycardia or cause transient AV block, which will help to diagnose the underlying atrial rhythm.

- In asthmatics or if adenosine is unsuccessful, consider verapamil 2.5–5 mg IV (do not use in patients receiving beta-blockers).

If all of this fails to terminate the tachycardia or has only a transient effect then try an AV node blocker:

- Digoxin load with 500 µg, two doses PO 4-hourly, then 250 µg PO OD, or…

- …flecainide 2 mg/kg IV over 30 minutes (monitor for AV block), or…

- …sotalol 80 mg PO BD.

Amiodarone can be used, but has a slow mode of onset orally and requires central IV infusion because of the risk of phlebitis.

You should also consider formal referral to an electrophysiologist.

Ventricular tachycardia (non-pulseless)

Confirm the ECG diagnosis. If you are unclear whether this is ventricular tachycardia or supraventricular tachycardia, try vagal manoeuvres or adenosine as before.

Treat the correctible factors!

- Aim for K^+ >4.5 mmol/L.

- Then, infuse IV Mg^{2+} 8 mmol/L over 15 minutes, then 72 mmol/L over 24 hours.

- Give amiodarone 300 mg IV over 30 minutes, then 900 mg over 24 hours via a large central vein.

Consider the following. But beware – they can all cause hypotension and aggravate heart failure!

- Beta-blockers (eg, metoprolol 25 mg PO TDS. This is short-acting, so has a quick wash-out if hypotension occurs).

- Flecainide 2 mg/kg IV over 30 minutes, maximum 150 mg.

- Procainamide 500–600 mg IV over 30 minutes, then 2–6 mg/minute IV.

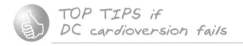

TOP TIPS if DC cardioversion fails

- Amiodarone IV 300 mg over 30 minutes, then 900 mg over 24 hours via a large central vein, or…

- …overdrive pacing.

Remember, pulseless ventricular tachycardia = ventricular fibrillation = *immediate defibrillation!*

6 Emergency Prescribing in Neurosurgery

Jane Ng

You shouldn't normally care for a neurosurgical patient in a non-specialist bed, but you might find yourself looking after such a patient while the referral is being made. The neurosurgical registrar will advise you with management. Remember to communicate any changes in the patient's neurological state to them, as a change in therapy might be required. You will only be asked to do a few things. Here are some top tips to help you.

Subarachnoid haemorrhage

By and large, SAHs are caused by the rupture of an intracranial artery. As a result:

- If you are conscious, it hurts!

- Raised ICP can arise from generalised cerebral oedema secondary to the insult and/or compression of the ventricular system by a resultant cerebral haematoma. This can reduce cerebral blood flow and cause cerebral ischaemia.

- Blood swilling around in the cerebrospinal fluid causes spasm of the large arteries in the base of the brain, resulting in even worse cerebral ischaemia.

- The vessel can rebleed.

Immediate management is therefore geared towards pain relief, maintaining cerebral perfusion (reducing ICP and limiting vasospasm) and reducing the risk of rebleeding.

Blood pressure control

Reactive arterial hypertension is common, and helps to maintain cerebral perfusion in the face of a raised ICP. But, too high a BP increases the risk of rebleeding, whilst too low a BP exacerbates cerebral ischaemia. Then there is the patient's usual BP to consider: someone who is usually hypertensive needs a higher BP than someone who is usually normotensive. So what BP *do* you aim for? As always, ask your neurosurgeon to guide you. Meanwhile, **Table 1** gives you some basic rules for BP control in SAH.

Spasm

Nimodipine is a (supposedly cerebroselective) calcium-channel antagonist. It saves lives after SAH by reducing spasm. Prescribe it as 60 mg PO 4-hourly. The BP might fall (as, in fact, nimodipine opens up all blood vessels). Treat this with colloid filling. If profound hypotension occurs after each dose, prescribe 30 mg PO 2-hourly instead.

Rebleeding

- Give all SAH patients regular stool softeners (eg, lactulose). Straining is a good way to have another bleed!

- *Do not* use NSAIDs for the pain.

- *Do not* use SC heparin as DVT prophylaxis. Use graded compression stockings instead.

Table 1. Action points for the management of SAH.

Do	Don't!
Have the patient 'head up 30 degrees'	Treat in order to get a 'normal BP' or be worried by a moderately raised BP. As a rule of thumb, aim for 20% higher than the baseline BP (if known)
Treat the pain! Start with paracetamol 1 g PO/NG/PR/IV QDS You can also use short-acting morphine sulphate (eg, morphine sulphate 5 mg PO 3-hourly PRN) or small doses (1–2 mg repeated doses) IV if the patient is vomiting. Small doses don't compromise neuroassessment	Use an NSAID – the anti-platelet effect increases the risk of rebleeding
Get HDU/ICU involved if you're at all concerned about the patient's consciousness or BP Gross hypertension should be treated with agents that can be 'switched off' (ie, avoid tablets) The intensivist will consider a short-acting IV anti-hypertensive such as labetalol (0.5–2 mg/minute to a maximum of 120 mg/hour) or glyceryl trinitrate (2–20 mg/hour). You should not have to do this	Reduce the BP too fast or too dramatically In general, do not use sublingual nifedipine as the response is fast, unpredictable, sustained and hard to reverse. Speak to the neurosurgeon!
AND REMEMBER FLUIDS! All SAH patients need enough fluid to counteract vasospasm. Keep your patient well hydrated! Giving fluid to an underfilled patient can help to bring the BP down (oddly enough!). The minimum fluid input should, in general, be 3 L of crystalloid in 24 hours. Avoid dextrose-containing solutions as these can worsen cerebral oedema. If the patient becomes hypotensive, fluid challenge them with colloid. If, in spite of this, the patient remains hypotensive, inotropes might be indicated: get HDU/ICU involved at this point!	

Bleeding and the brain

In any cerebral bleed, or where one is likely:

- *Do not* give warfarin. If the patient is on warfarin, reverse it (see **Section 5, Chapter 1**).

- *Avoid* heparin DVT prophylaxis: use graded compression stockings instead.

- *Avoid* NSAIDs.

- Consider ulcer prophylaxis, as stress ulceration is common.

Steroids and neurosurgery

Steroids reduce swelling around tumours, relieving cord compression and lowering ICP. They also reduce neuronal swelling associated with cauda equina compression secondary to a prolapsed disc. Prescribe a one-off loading dose of dexamethasone 8 mg PO. Follow this with a regular prescription of dexamethasone 4 mg PO QDS. This is a large dose of steroid and will usually lead to a dramatic improvement in the patient's symptoms and signs. If the patient is with you for a while, the dose can be reduced as the patient tolerates, leaving them on a smaller baseline dose (eg, dexamethasone 4 mg PO BD).

Steroid use in acute spinal injury is a contentious issue. Initial trials showed that methylprednisolone given within 8 hours of injury was beneficial. However, more recent data have challenged this. Moreover, these trials suggest that steroid use might in fact be harmful. Ask the neurosurgeon what to do.

Mannitol and neurosurgery

Mannitol is an osmotic diuretic. It can reduce ICP and, in certain cases, is a useful temporary holding measure until the patient can be delivered to a neurosurgical unit for a definitive operative procedure. Only give on the instruction of a neurosurgeon.

Mannitol methods

Mannitol 20% comes in 500 mL bottles, which contain 100 g of drug.

- Dose: 20% mannitol 0.5–1.0 g/kg IV over 15–20 minutes.

- In practice: *20% mannitol 200 mL IV over 20 minutes.*

- Only repeat if instructed: it can paradoxically increase ICP.

- It will cause an osmotic diuresis. Catheterise! Watch electrolytes! Beware dehydration!

Anti-convulsants and neurosurgery

Remember to ask about anti-convulsants. A fit is a very good way of making a brain injury worse by increasing brain metabolism, causing hypoxia (with the fit) and raising ICP (with all the thrashing around). Phenytoin is often used (see **Section 7, Chapter 4**). Prophylactic anti-epileptics are rarely indicated.

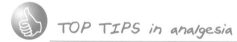 TOP TIPS *in analgesia*

- Codeine works by being converted to morphine. Five to 10% of people can't do this at all and about 30% do it badly. *Codeine is weak and its effects unreliable.*

- If giving an opioid, the dose needed will vary from patient to patient – so dilute it down (eg, morphine 10 mg in 20 mL saline) and give it mL by mL until you have the effect you want.

- *Do not* use NSAIDs in patients where you want clotting to work properly – like those with SAH!

Massive Pulmonary Embolism

7

Rob Shulman

(with acknowledgement to *UCLH Guidelines for Medical Emergencies*, edited by Adrian Wagg and Carolyn Gates)

It is currently being debated whether IV heparin alone is sufficient to treat a massive PE or whether thrombolysis is also needed. In general, thrombolysis might be preferred in those with significant right heart strain or circulatory embarrassment.

IV heparin

Start heparin bolus and infusion (see **Section 5, Chapter 2**), but stop before thrombolysis is started (see below).

Thrombolysis

Ideally, the APTT ratio should be <1.5 before thrombolysis starts, but do not delay if the condition appears to be immediately life-threatening.

- For stable massive PE patients, give a 10 mg IV bolus of alteplase over 1–2 minutes, then 90 mg over 2 hours (to a maximum total dose of 1.5 mg/kg if <65 kg body weight).

- For patients who are rapidly deteriorating and in whom cardiac arrest is imminent, or who have an in-house cardiac arrest, give a 50 mg IV bolus of alteplase and reassess after 30 minutes.

- Having completed the alteplase infusion, wait 2.5 hours, then start unfractionated heparin (see **Section 5, Chapter 2**). Ideally, the APTT ratio should be <2.0. Aim for an APTT ratio between 1.5 and 2.5.

- Start warfarin on day 3–7 of heparin therapy and continue until the INR is in the desired range for two consecutive days, with at least 5 days' overlap.

If you need to restore coagulation pre-operatively, give IV aprotinin 500,000–1,000,000 KIU (50–100 mL) over 10–20 minutes (consider the patient's weight), then an IV infusion of 200,000–500,000 KIU/hour (20–50 mL/hour). Remember that surgical thrombectomy is now rarely performed.

Management of bleeding during thrombolysis

Bleeding can occur even when coagulation screening tests are normal. It is essential that patients are regularly monitored for clinical signs of bleeding. If internal bleeding is suspected, consider whether the infusion of thrombolytic therapy should be stopped and investigations undertaken.

- For minor, local bleeding – apply sustained pressure.

- For more serious bleeding – stop the infusion of alteplase and heparin (depleted fibrinogen, factor V and factor VIII should be restored within 12–24 hours).

- For severe, life-threatening bleeding – discontinue alteplase and heparin. Administer IV aprotinin immediately, as above, continuing the infusion until bleeding stops. Alternatively, administer tranexamic acid 1 g IV over 15 minutes, repeated 8-hourly as necessary. Administer FFP and/or cryoprecipitate to replenish depleted clotting factors, depending on the coagulation screen.

Electrolyte and Metabolic Emergencies

8

Jane Ng

Electrolyte and metabolic abnormalities can present insidiously (eg, weakness with prolonged hypokalaemia) or kill rapidly (eg, rapid-onset hyperkalaemia). Worse, there might be little warning, with the patient looking 'pretty well'. Do not be deceived! And never delay in responding!

General rules

Avoiding trouble

Most trouble is iatrogenic – and much of it is due to IV fluid therapy. This often causes electrolyte imbalance, so assess the patient's hydration status accurately and look at urea, creatinine and electrolytes. Then prescribe the right choice of IV fluid at the right dose and reassess regularly. Is the patient dry? Overloaded? Passing urine? Hyponatraemic?

Decide how often you should check the bloods. Hourly if severe hyperkalaemia? Twice daily if vomiting or with a high-output fistula? Daily if NBM and on an IV infusion? Weekly if 'long-term and stable'?

Managing trouble

If you spot a problem:

- Decide how *urgent* it is. A potassium level that's up from 4.2 to 5.4 mmol/L over 24 hours might need a repeat check (to confirm) now, and again later to monitor any trend. If the potassium is 8.2 mmol/L and a repeat check on the gas machine says 9.3 mmol/L then this is an emergency *now! Right this second!*

- Stop *causing* the problem. Adjust the IV fluid rate or nature. Examine the drug chart and cross off any obvious culprits, eg, the hyperkalaemic on ACE inhibitors or spironolactone (or both!).

- Stop the *patient* causing the problem. Are they abusing laxatives? Are they eating bananas and cheese when in incipient renal failure?

- Identify any *disease* causing the problem. What's the electrolyte content of that fistula fluid? Could they be Addisonian?

Specific management

Getting high!

Hyperkalaemia

A high plasma potassium (K^+) level needs treating (see **Table 2**). The urgency or imperative for this varies with the speed of the rise – a slow rise to 8.2 mmol/L over a few months isn't as worrying as a rise to 6.6 mmol/L over a day. In general, be worried if K^+ is rising fast or is already >6.5 mmol/L.

Table 2. Options for the treatment of hyperkalaemia.

The three elements to treatment	Prescribe
Cardioprotection High K$^+$ destabilises cell membrane potential. Cardiac cells are particularly susceptible, and cardiac arrest can ensue	10 mL 10% calcium gluconate or calcium chloride IV over 2 minutes Repeat if there are any subsequent ECG signs consistent with hyperkalaemia. This might be hazardous to those on digoxin
Lowering plasma levels by pushing K$^+$ into the cells Insulin pushes K$^+$ into cells. Concurrent glucose prevents hypoglycaemia	10 units of human soluble insulin (Actrapid) added to 50 mL of 50% glucose IV to run over 15 minutes This lowers K$^+$ by 1 mmol/L in 30 minutes. Follow-up by running another similar infusion, but over 1 hour Alternatively, nebulised salbutamol is highly effective (and some say better)
Binding K$^+$ Pushing K$^+$ into cells is a quick fix. Binding K$^+$, promoting its excretion, is more definitive	Calcium polystyrene sulfonate (Calcium Resonium®) 15 g PO TDS Always prescribe with lactulose (at least 10 mL TDS) as it is extremely constipating

Then:

Repeat bloods at about 2 hours. Call ahead to the lab – let them know that it's urgent. Using the blood gas machine (if available to you) is generally faster.

If the plasma K$^+$ remains >6.5 mmol/L, consult a senior doctor or the renal team – dialysis might be indicated.

Here's one last holding measure that you might be asked to try: 100 mL of 8.4% sodium bicarbonate IV over 10–20 minutes given through a large vein, or 500 mL of 1.26% sodium bicarbonate IV over 1 hour. Bicarbonate also pushes K$^+$ into cells.

Table 3. Options for the treatment of hypercalcaemia

The three elements to treatment	Prescribe
Rehydrate	
These patients are almost always dry!	Appropriate IV fluids
Promote urinary calcium excretion	
Once rehydrated, continue IV fluids, encouraging diuresis. Also, loop diuretics cause hypocalcaemia as well as diuresis	Furosemide 20 mg IV OD
Limit endogenous Ca^{2+} production	
Inhibit osteoclastic activity with bisphosphonates	Pamidronate IV at a maximum concentration of 30 mg in 125 mL of 0.9% sodium chloride and a maximum rate of 60 mg/hour
This is the most effective way of lowering Ca^{2+}, but takes 1–2 days to take effect	
Maximum effects are seen by day 5 and last 2–4 weeks	

Note:	
Plasma Ca^{2+} (mmol/L)	**Pamidronate dose (mg)**
<3.0	15–30
3.0–3.5	30–60
3.5–4.0	60–90
>4.0	90

Then: once plasma Ca^{2+} starts to fall, usually by day 2, switch to oral fluids, aiming for at least 2 L/day.

Hypercalcaemia

A plasma calcium (Ca^{2+}) level >3.5 mmol/L generally needs urgent treatment (see **Table 3**). Again, the imperative varies with the absolute level and speed of rise.

Hyperthyroidism

Thyrotoxic crisis, thyroid storm (see **Table 4**).

Table 4. Options for the treatment of hyperthyroidism.

The three elements to treatment	Prescribe
Prevent the synthesis of thyroid hormone	Carbimazole 15–25 mg/day PO/NG QDS or propylthiouracil 150–300 mg/day PO/NG QDS
Block the function of the thyroid gland by flooding it with iodine	Sodium iodide 1–2 g IV over 3–5 minutes or IV infusion over 8–24 hours or Lugol's solution 0.3 mL PO/NG TDS
Treat symptoms	Propranolol 1 mg IV over 1 minute (repeat if needed up to 10 times at 2-minute intervals) or propranolol 40 mg PO/NG QDS

Then:

After 5 days, reduce the carbimazole to 20 mg PO/NG TDS.

Adjust this dose according to response.

After 10 days, stop propranolol and iodine.

Feeling low...

Dangerously low levels of electrolytes and hormones are treated by replacement. The actual amount you give will depend on the severity of depletion and the response of the patient – ask your registrar! **Table 5** shows the available preparations.

Table 5. Options for hormonal and electrolyte supplementation.

	Parenteral replacement	Enteral replacement
Potassium	Available in 20 mmol/L bags If you want to give ≥60 mmol/L of K⁺ then you need central access and ECG monitoring	Sando-K®: 12 mmol/L of K⁺ per tablet Slow K⁺ (containing 8 mmol/tablet) can cause oesophageal irritation, so tell your patient to take the tablets in an upright position, drinking water before and after
Magnesium	Mg^{2+} encourages K⁺ uptake Prescribe 20 mmol/L of Mg^{2+} as a one-off when replacing K⁺ Aim for an overall plasma Mg^{2+} of 1 mmol/L	Magnesium glycerophosphate, 4 mmol of Mg^{2+} per tablet
Sodium	Familiarise yourself with how many mmol/L of Na⁺ there are in all of the different types of fluids available In situations where parenteral sodium replacement is required (eg, hyponatraemic seizures), the patient should be on the ICU	The use of oral Na⁺ supplementation is controversial. An example of use is in neurosurgical patients with cerebral salt wasting Na⁺ supplements are available as Slow Sodium® in 10 mmol/L tablets, prescribed at 4–8 tablets/day
Calcium	In hypocalcaemic tetany, parenteral calcium is given as 10 mL of 10% calcium chloride or calcium gluconate (2.25 mmol), followed by an infusion of 40 mL (9 mmol) daily	A large selection of oral calcium supplements is available. A common preparation is Calcichew®, which contains 12.6 mmol of Ca^{2+} per tablet.
Glucose	For hypoglycaemic coma, 50 mL of 20% glucose can be given IV Alternatively, glucagon 1 mg can be given IV, IM or SC. This is useful if IV access cannot be established	Hypoglycaemia is rapidly treated with 10–20 g glucose. This is equivalent to 2 teaspoons of sugar, 3 sugar lumps, one GlucoGel gel ampoule, 200 mL milk, 50–55 mL non-diet Lucozade, 90 mL cola or 15 mL Ribena Original (see **Chapter 3**)

Table 5. *Continued*

	Parenteral replacement	**Enteral replacement**
Thyroid hormone	Liothyronine sodium is used for severe hypothyroid states. Seek specialist advice in these cases Remember to give a shot of steroid when treating severe hypothyroidism – treating hypothyroidism can unmask life-threatening hypoadrenalism	Levothyroxine is usually commenced at 50–100 μg, then titrated up to a maintenance dose of 100–200 μg in steps of 50 μg every 3–4 weeks Dose reduction is required in cardiac and elderly patients
Steroid hormones	In acute adrenocortical insufficiency, IV hydrocortisone is given in doses of 100 mg every 6–8 hours in a sodium chloride infusion	In Addison's disease or following adrenalectomy, hydrocortisone is given at 20–30 mg PO daily. The dose is usually divided 2/3–1/3, with the larger dose given in the morning, thereby consistent with the physiological circadian rhythm of cortisol. Glucocorticoid therapy is also supplemented with fludrocortisone 50–300 μg daily With pituitary deficiency, the fludrocortisone is not necessary as the renin–angiotensin system that regulates its release remains intact

9 Respiratory Emergencies

Jane Ng

Patients in respiratory distress are frightening. Revise your British Thoracic Society guidelines on the management of asthma and COPD. Here are some top tips on what drugs need to be prescribed and how to prescribe them.

Remember: nearly all breathless patients (bar those with massive PE) are better sitting upright. Before putting pen to paper, sit the patient up! This optimises their ventilatory capacity and will also optimise inhaled drug delivery.

Then, oxygen

In asthma, *always* give the maximum oxygen possible. With a face mask and a rebreather bag at a flow rate of 10 L/minute, you can achieve an FiO_2 of approximately 0.9.

Some COPD patients rely on their hypoxic drive to breathe. However, in the emergency setting, it might not be hypercapnia but *hypoxia* that kills. In the absence of signs of normal CO_2 retention (high bicarbonate, $PaCO_2$ elevated out of keeping with more modest acidosis), give high-flow oxygen to the acutely unwell patient – and watch them closely and repeat the gases in 20–30 minutes. Increasing drowsiness or rising $PaCO_2$ might suggest that you need to reduce the FiO_2 – or just that the patient was going to tire anyway and now needs mechanical ventilatory support.

Table 6. Optimising the effect of nebulised salbutamol and ipratropium.

	Salbutamol	Ipratropium bromide
Dose	2.5–5 mg	500 µg
Frequency	Give stat and again after 15–30 minutes if the patient is not improving If the patient is improving, give 4-hourly, with a PRN dose 2-hourly	Give if life-threatening features are present If the patient is not improving, give 6-hourly until the patient improves
Mode	Nebuliser	Nebuliser

Inhaled bronchodilators

Salbutamol is the first-line inhaled bronchodilator used, then ipratropium bromide (see **Table 6**).

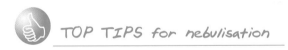

TOP TIPS for nebulisation

- Ensure that the patient is sitting up, thereby increasing airway patency.

- The driving gas can either be oxygen or air. *Always* use oxygen in patients with asthma. *Beware* in those with COPD!

- Ask the patient to breathe through their mouth, preventing nasal deposition of the drug.

- Ask the patient if they would prefer a mouthpiece or face mask. Ipratropium bromide is preferably given via a mouthpiece as this prevents ocular deposition and glaucoma.

- Salbutamol and ipratropium bromide can be mixed and nebulised together.

- If the patient isn't tolerating nebulisers, try a spacer device: 1 puff of salbutamol from a metered dose inhaler = 100 µg (ie, 5 mg dose = 50 puffs). Perhaps give 10 puffs into the spacer, asking the patient to take 10 deep breaths, then repeat four more times. This is a good trick for kids, who might not like nebulisers.

Intravenous bronchodilators

Theophylline

Theophylline is indicated in acute asthma when life-threatening features are present or if the patient has not responded to initial therapy. Its IV form is aminophylline, which is available in 250 mg (10 mL) ampoules. See **Section 7, Chapter 4** for dosing and monitoring.

How many COPD patients have you ever met who are lean, non-smokers and taking no other tablets (all of these factors affect theophylline therapy)? Not many? And how do you feel about using an emergency drug when you might have no idea that the levels are therapeutic for over a day?

For these reasons, many have abandoned aminophylline and now prefer to use IV salbutamol.

Salbutamol

IV salbutamol is indicated in asthma when life-threatening features are present or if the patient has not responded to initial therapy. Prescribe salbutamol 250 µg IV over 20 minutes. Infusions can run at 1–20 µg/minute, according to response. The half-life is short, so increased infusion causes a rapid response and toxic effects quickly die away when rates are reduced. Being a selective receptor agonist, general side-effects (eg, tremor, agitation) are also far fewer!

Corticosteroids

Some data indicate that response can be quite quick so, at presentation, prescribe *both* hydrocortisone 200 mg IV and prednisolone 40 mg PO. Continue prednisolone 40 mg PO OD or hydrocortisone 200 mg IV BD thereafter. If sustained therapy isn't required, the dose can be weaned over 5 days.

Newer therapies

Magnesium chloride can be added for severe asthmatics: 2 g in 50 mL of 0.9% sodium chloride IV over 30 minutes. This is usually given as a one-off.

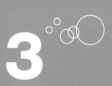

3

Gastrointestinal System

1. Practical Prescribing in
   General Gastroenterology   89

2. Constipation in the Adult Patient   92

3. Nausea and Vomiting   95

4. Safe Prescribing in Liver Disease   97

5. Practical Total Parenteral Nutrition   99

Practical Prescribing in General Gastroenterology

1

Caroline Green and Rebecca White

GI complaints are common. Here are some general rules to help you manage them.

Dyspepsia (non-ulcer)

Stop! First, check that the diagnosis isn't more serious. If it really is dyspepsia then, before wading in with treatment, determine any possible cause (eg, NSAIDs, delayed gastric emptying, caffeine intake) – and manage appropriately.

If no removable cause is present, start the patient on a 4-week course of a PPI (eg, omeprazole 10–20 mg OD, lansoprazole 15–30 mg OD) and then reassess the symptoms. Treatment regimens for reducing stomach acid secretion in various illnesses are given in **Table 1**.

Diarrhoea

First, resuscitate the patient (fluids *and* electrolytes might be depleted). Oral resuscitation should be your first option, if possible. Then, identify the cause (eg, cancer, infection, colitis) and treat appropriately. *Always* check (especially in the elderly) that it isn't really faecal impaction with over-flow.

Table 1. Reducing stomach acid secretion.

Disorder	Regimen
Dyspepsia (non-ulcer)	If no removable cause, prescribe a 4-week course of a PPI then reassess
Gastro-oesophageal reflux disease	Prescribe a 4- to 8-week course of a PPI then reduce to the lowest dose that controls the patient's symptoms
Duodenal ulcers	Eradicate *H. pylori* [a] If ulceration is still present, continue with another 4-week course of a PPI If symptoms continue, repeat the 4-week course of a PPI then reduce to the lowest dose that controls the patient's symptoms
Gastric ulcers	Eradicate *H. pylori* [a] Continue PPI treatment for another 8 weeks Review endoscopy results at 6–8 weeks to determine whether to continue treatment
Acute GI bleed from an ulcer	Having endoscoped the patient, your gastroenterologist might ask you to prescribe a PPI infusion (eg, omeprazole 80 mg loading dose then 8 mg/hour for 72 hours)

[a] *H. pylori* eradication therapy: this is a 1-week oral course of three drugs (one PPI and two antibiotics). The actual antibiotics will depend on local policy and penicillin allergies. Example: omeprazole 20 mg BD, amoxicillin 1 g BD (or metronidazole 400 mg BD), clarithromycin 500 mg BD.

If anti-diarrhoeal agents are required, use:

- codeine phosphate 30 mg PO TDS/QDS, or…

- …loperamide 4 mg PO initially, then 2 mg after each loose stool for up to 5 days (a maximum of 16 mg daily)

Make sure that you check with someone more senior first – these drugs should not be used in over-flow diarrhoea caused by faecal impaction or in infective diarrhoea.

High-output stomas

See **Section 6, Chapter 1**.

Inflammatory bowel disease

This is a specialist area – but here are some basics to think about whilst you wait for the gastroenterology registrar to review.

Treatment of acute exacerbations (in pre-diagnosed patients) includes:

- fluid resuscitation

- thromboprophylaxis with LMWH SC

- hydrocortisone 100 mg IV QDS

- prednisolone 20 mg PR OD for predominantly left-sided disease

- continuing or commencing an aminosalicylate; the precise preparation will depend on where the disease is (follow specialist advice)

In the unwell inflammatory bowel disease patient:

Check the drug history. Drugs such as azathioprine, mercaptopurine and methotrexate are commonly used in inflammatory bowel disease. Check FBC for neutropenia and LFTs for any abnormalities.

- Azathioprine is usually given at a dose of 2–3 mg/kg/day OD.

- Methotrexate is usually given as 15–25 mg PO/SC once-weekly. The patient usually also takes folic acid, but only on 5 days of the week.

2 Constipation in the Adult Patient

Olivia Hameer

A common scenario! A *DIPER* will prevent you from falling between stools!

Diagnosis

Find out what is normal for your patient – three bowel movements a day or three a week? Constipation isn't necessarily lack of frequency: it might be the passing of hard, painful faeces or difficulty in full evacuation.

Identify a cause

Look for all the *D*s:

- *D*isease (eg, endocrine, metabolic or neurological disturbances)

- *D*isability (immobility)

- *D*ietary change (never underestimate the effect of hospital food!)

- *D*ehydration

- *D*rug treatment (eg, antacids containing aluminium, anti-cholinergics, iron salts, opioid analgesics including co-proxamol, phenothiazines, tricyclic anti-depressants, verapamil, anti-Parkinsonian drugs, diuretics, amiodarone, clonidine, lithium, NSAIDs, anti-diarrhoeals)

Table 2. Laxative classes with recommended initial doses.

Type of laxative	Example
Bulk forming	Ispaghula husk (Fybogel), 1 sachet PO BD
Stimulant	Senna, 2–4 tablets PO nocte
	Sodium docusate, 100 mg PO BD/TDS
	Co-danthramer, 5–10 mL PO nocte
Softener	Arachis oil, 1 enema PR stat
Osmotic	Lactulose, 10–15 mL PO BD
	Glycerin, 1 suppository PR OD
	Phosphate, 1 enema PR OD
	Sodium citrate (Micolette Micro-enema®), 1 enema PR OD
Possible regimens for:	
Acute constipation	Stimulant laxative
Chronic constipation	Osmotic or bulk-forming laxative
Opioid-induced constipation	Stimulant laxative
Terminal disease	Stimulant laxative

Prompt the patient

Encourage your patient to:

- eat fresh fruit and vegetables, wholegrain breads and coarse bran

- drink 2 L of fluids per day

- exercise

Elect to prescribe a laxative

This is not the first step in the management of constipation! If you have to use drugs, use the least number of drugs for the least amount of time (see **Table 2**).

Review the patient

Stool charts should be kept. A fluid balance chart is also helpful. Review laxative therapy regularly and discontinue when it's no longer needed. Laxative dependence should be avoided!

Nausea and Vomiting

Simon Noble and Clare Turner

Choose an anti-emetic according to the mechanism of vomiting (see **Table 3**). Is the cause of the nausea central, vestibular or poison-related, or due to gastric outflow obstruction? Imagine that you go out for a heavy night of drinking…

- You drink 10 pints in a couple of hours. You feel sick, have a large-volume vomit and feel better. Mechanism of vomiting: *gastric distension*. You need a prokinetic (eg, metoclopramide, domperidone).

- Avoiding beers this time! You drink shots all night, so less volume. At the end of the night you feel sick. Mechanism of nausea: poisoning. You need a *centrally acting drug* (eg, haloperidol [D_2 antagonist], cyclizine [H_2 antagonist and anti-cholinergic]).

- You finally settle. Friends get you into a taxi. You are sick. Mechanism: *vestibular disturbance*. You need something to work on the *ACh/H_2 receptors* (eg, cyclizine, prochlorperazine).

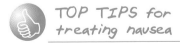

TOP TIPS for treating nausea

- Ondansetron only hits one receptor and causes severe constipation.

- Haloperidol and cyclizine make a good combination, covering many receptors.

Table 3. Anti-emetic drugs, mechanisms of action and their clinical uses.

Drug	Mechanism of action	Clinical use
Metoclopramide	Prokinetic, weak D_2 antagonist	Gastric outflow obstruction
		Upper GI bleed
		Liver metastases
		Cancer at the head of the pancreas
Haloperidol	Good central anti-emetic effect (D_2 antagonist)	Poison-related nausea
		Hypercalcaemia
		Uraemia
		Nausea secondary to antibiotics and opioids
Cyclizine	ACh/H_2 (central acting)	Raised ICP
		Central causes
		Motion sickness/ vestibular problems
Ondansetron/ granisetron	$5HT_3$ antagonist (very constipating)	Chemotherapy-induced nausea

- Never give metoclopramide and cyclizine together. The anti-muscarinic effect of cyclizine blocks the prokinetic effect of metoclopramide, rendering it as much help as a chocolate fireguard.

- The 'Domestos' of anti-emetics is levomepromazine (Nozinan®). However, it's not regularly used because it's sedating. Talk to the palliative care team before using it.

Safe Prescribing in Liver Disease

Caroline Green and Rebecca White

Liver disease can affect both drug choice and dosing.

- *Jaundice:* high bilirubin levels displace highly protein-bound drugs such as metronidazole and phenytoin. Doses might need to be reduced (see **Section 7, Chapter 4** for phenytoin dosing in low albumin states).

- *Cholestasis* or a *hepatitic picture* with impaired clotting suggests an acute effect on synthetic function. Drugs metabolised by the liver should be avoided where possible.

- *Cirrhosis* causes a reduction in the 'first-pass' effect as the blood is shunted around the liver, not through it. In real terms, this means that some drugs will have a much higher bioavailability and a longer half-life.

In addition, try to avoid drugs that cause abnormal LFTs and cloud the clinical picture (eg, statins, flucloxacillin, fluconazole; co-amoxiclav causes a cholestatic picture). If in doubt, consult your pharmacist!

Table 4 looks at the end-stage liver disease patient as an example of drug prescribing.

Acute alcoholic admission? See **Section 1, Chapter 8**.

Table 4. Drug options for the management of the end-stage liver disease patient.

Drug option	Treatment
Analgesia	Paracetamol 500 mg PO QDS (dose is half the usual)
	Avoid NSAIDs. They increase the risk of a GI bleed and cause fluid retention
	Use opioids with caution: even small doses can cause profound and prolonged encephalopathy, and precipitate decompensation
Diuretic therapy	Used to aid the treatment of ascites
	Conventionally, spironolactone 100–200 mg PO OD. Adjust the dose every 48 hours
	Other diuretics promote a too-aggressive diuresis, leading to decompensation
Clotting agents	With a rising INR, give vitamin K 10 mg IV (if bleeding) or PO (without bleeding), usually for 3 days, then reassess
	In the setting of acute bleeding, give FFP/cryoprecipitate
Anti-pruritic	Nothing works well. Try:
	• colestyramine 4 g PO BD (you will need to adjust the doses of all other drugs as this can affect absorption)
	• menthol in aqueous cream can help to soothe the itching
	Avoid sedating anti-histamines, which exacerbate encephalopathy
Laxatives	Lactulose 20 mL PO BD/TDS is the drug of choice. It discourages the proliferation of ammonia-producing organisms, thereby helping the treatment of encephalopathy
Anti-seizure medication	Phenytoin
	It is imperative to monitor levels (see **Section 7, Chapter 4**)
Treating bleeding oesophageal varices	Terlipressin 2 mg IV 4- to 6-hourly until bleeding is controlled (for up to 72 hours)

Practical Total Parenteral Nutrition

Rebecca White

Two golden facts

Fact 1. One in five patients admitted to UK hospitals is significantly malnourished, and vastly more will become so.

Fact 2. Malnutrition kills – but in ways that you won't spot (eg, wound infection, susceptibility to infections).

So feed your patients!

Two golden rules

Rule 1. Involve a dietician *early* – as soon as you suspect malnutrition or the risk of malnutrition.

Rule 2. If the gut works, use it! If the patient cannot swallow, place a fine-bore feeding tube. Endoscopists, surgeons and radiologists can help you with this.

What about parenteral nutrition?

Seek advice! Commonly, you will just be asked to sign the prescription. Before putting pen to paper, think sic*K*ly – you need to *K*now…

- …the indication for parenteral nutrition. Remember: parenteral nutrition is never an emergency (except in children, and experts will always manage these patients). Low albumin does not usually indicate that the patient is malnourished – it is usually an indicator of how sick they are. Parenteral nutrition is *not* a cure for low albumin

- …recent biochemistry, including Ca^{2+}, Mg^{2+}, PO_4^{2-}

- …recent weight

- …if a fluid restriction has been set

- …any medical complications that will affect requirements (eg, renal, liver, cardiovascular disease)

- …what venous access the patient has/requires for parenteral nutrition

Then, Know what's in a bag and how much

A bag can contain:

- calories as glucose and fat

- protein as basic amino acids (expressed as grams of nitrogen)

- water

- electrolytes (Na^+, K^+, Ca^{2+}, Mg^{2+}, PO_4^{2-}, Cl^-)

- vitamins and trace elements

Lastly, Know about re-feeding syndrome in sick, malnourished patients

Here, a surge in insulin levels causes a rapid drop in K^+, PO_4^{2-} and Mg^{2+} levels, which can have severe clinical consequences. Avoid by starting parenteral nutrition at a low rate and building it up – and monitor electrolytes daily.

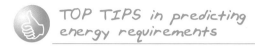

TOP TIPS in predicting energy requirements

Healthcare professionals working in this area use standard equations to predict energy requirements. These are usually related to body mass: for underweight and normal weight patients you should use actual bodyweight, but for obese patients you should use *ideal* body weight. In broad terms, prescriptions boil down to:

- calories: 20–30 kcal/kg/day

- nitrogen: 0.17 g/kg/day

- fluid: approximately 30 mL/kg/day (ensure any unnecessary fluids are discontinued)

Remember: more isn't better! Over-feeding is the cause of most complications.

4

Central Nervous System

1.	Analgesia	105
2.	Patient-controlled Analgesia	114
3.	Epidural Analgesia	117
4.	Prescribing in Palliative Care	121
5.	Fit for a Fit: Adults with Seizures	126
6.	Insomnia	131

Analgesia

Suparna Bali

(See also **Chapter 4** of this section.)

Inadequate analgesia, or the use of the wrong drug doses or combinations, will diminish your patients' quality of life and slow their recovery. So learn the concepts of basic analgesia and *get advice early* (eg, from your hospital's 'pain team').

The World Health Organisation analgesic ladder

Step 3

Strong opioid for moderate to severe pain (eg, morphine) + non-opioid

Step 2

Weak opioid for mild to moderate pain + non-opioid

Step 1

Non-opioid (eg, paracetamol and/or NSAID)

TOP TIPS when using the analgesic ladder

- Start at the bottom 'rung' with paracetamol or NSAIDs. If this is ineffective, try them together.

- If this fails, move up the ladder – *do not* add another drug from the same class!

- Regular administration of analgesia is more effective than PRN dosing. In addition, doses of analgesics that are given regularly to keep the pain away will be lower than PRN doses given to treat the pain when it returns.

- Whichever drug you choose, start with the lowest possible dose and increase according to response.

- Avoid using more than one opioid at a time.

- Use the minimum dose necessary to achieve the required pain relief – this will differ from patient to patient and from day to day.

The ladder has no top 'rung' as there is no upper limit for strong opioids. However, if the patient does need high doses then the cause of the pain must be re-investigated.

Drug choices

Table 1 gives examples of step 1 and 2 analgesics, the usual doses they are prescribed at and some advantages and disadvantages of their use. Bear in mind that you might come across the odd patient who is an exception to these general prescribing rules.

Table 1. Analgesics used in steps 1 and 2 of the pain ladder. *Continued overleaf.*

Drug	Dose	Plus points	Downsides
Non-opioids			
Paracetamol	1 g PO/IV/ PR QDS	Same dose for all routes	Caution in liver/ renal disease
Ibuprofen[a]	1.2–1.8 g PO in 3–4 divided doses daily Can be increased to a max. of 2.4 g daily	Anti-inflammatory Analgesic and anti-pyretic effects	Caution in renal, cardiac or hepatic impairment Caution if on concurrent anti-coagulation Contraindicated in patients with active peptic ulceration
Diclofenac[a]	75–150 mg PO/PR in 2–3 divided doses (max. 150 mg in 24 hours) Can be given IM, but only for 2 days	As for ibuprofen	As for ibuprofen
Opioids			
Codeine[b]	30–60 mg PO every 4–6 hours or 30–60 mg PO/IM every 4–6 hours	For mild to moderate pain	Caution in renal/liver impairment May not work for 5–10% of patients Can cause constipation

[a] NSAIDs (based on *BNF* recommendation): your choice of NSAID will depend on what is available in your hospital. Base your choice on the relative GI safety, tolerability and efficacy relevant to your patient's clinical situation. The risk of GI toxicity is higher in the elderly population, with azapropazone posing the greatest risk and ibuprofen the lowest. Piroxicam, ketoprofen, indomethacin, naproxen and diclofenac are considered to be intermediate risks. *Never use more than one NSAID at a time!*

[b] Codeine is metabolised to morphine – but 5–10% of people do not metabolise codeine at all due to the lack of a specific enzyme.

Table 1. *Continued.*

Drug	Dose	Plus points	Downsides
Dihydrocodeine[b]	30 mg PO every 4–6 hours or up to 50 mg IM/deep SC 4–6 hourly if required	Analgesic efficacy similar to codeine, but less constipating	Caution in renal/liver impairment Can cause constipation
Tramadol	50–100 mg PO/IM every 4–6 hours	Acts at serotonergic receptors as well as opioid receptors, so useful for neuropathic pain Less constipating than codeine	Caution in renal/liver impairment Contraindicated in uncontrolled epilepsy Can cause hallucinations More expensive

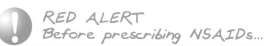

RED ALERT
Before prescribing NSAIDs...

Before prescribing NSAIDs, check for:

- hypersensitivity and allergic reactions to aspirin or NSAIDs (these are absolute contraindications!)

- asthma

- a history of GI problems

- renal impairment

- liver impairment

- bleeding tendencies

Compound analgesics

Compound analgesics are used for mild to moderate pain. They contain paracetamol (or aspirin) combined with an opioid (eg, codeine, dihydrocodeine). **Table 2** shows the content of the more common preparations.

Table 2. Constituents of some commonly prescribed compound analgesics.

Analgesic	Tablet constituents
Co-codamol 8/500	Codeine phosphate 8 mg + paracetamol 500 mg
Co-codamol 30/500 (eg, Solpadol®, Tylex®)	Codeine phosphate 30 mg + paracetamol 500 mg
Co-dydramol	Dihydrocodeine 10 mg + paracetamol 500 mg

 RED ALERT for compound analgesics

- The maximum dose of paracetamol is 1 g QDS. Check that this is not being exceeded with these compound preparations.

- Even with the low dose of opioid in these compound preparations, susceptible groups (eg, older patients) will be at risk of side-effects.

- Compound preparations do not allow you to titrate the doses of the constituent drugs separately – this can hamper optimal acute pain management.

Opioid analgesics

Opioids offer excellent analgesia for moderate to severe pain. They can be administered by several different routes, and their use should be tailored to the patient's needs.

The idea that 'morphine derivatives' are only reserved for cancer patients is wrong! Yes, there are potential side effects (eg, nausea, vomiting, constipation, pruritus, tolerance, addiction) and large doses can cause respiratory depression and hypotension – but this should *not* deter you from prescribing them where indicated. Choice of opioid is important and care should be taken when performing conversions (see **Table 3**).

Table 3. Opioid conversion table.

Drug	Dose	Approximate equivalent oral morphine dose	Approximate conversion factor to oral morphine
Buprenorphine	200 µg S/L	12 mg	×60
Codeine phosphate	60 mg PO	6 mg	×0.1
Dihydrocodeine	60 mg PO	6 mg	×0.1
Dihydrocodeine	50 mg SC/IM	15 mg	×0.3
Diamorphine	10 mg IV/SC/IM	30 mg	×3
Hydromorphone	2.6 mg PO	20 mg	×7.5
Methadone	PO	Seek expert advice	Seek expert advice
Morphine sulphate (immediate-release)	10 mg PO	10 mg	×1
Morphine sulphate (modified-release) MST®	30 mg PO	30 mg	×1
Morphine sulphate	5 mg SC/IM	10 mg	×2
Morphine sulphate	5 mg IV	10–15 mg	×2–3
Oxycodone	10 mg PO	20 mg	×2
Pethidine	50 mg PO	6.25 mg	×0.125
Pethidine	100 mg SC/IM	25 mg	×0.25

Note: These are approximate conversions; other reference sources may differ.
Source: Adapted from University College London Hospitals Formulary, 2002.

TOP TIPS when prescribing opioids

- Morphine and diamorphine are the opioids of choice for severe pain.

- *Always* prescribe an anti-emetic alongside the opioid (eg, cyclizine 50 mg PO/IV/SC TDS) – and give it *before* the first dose of opioid...

- …and also add a laxative (eg, two senna tablets nocte).

- Pruritus can be relieved with an anti-histamine
  (eg, chlorpheniramine).

- Patients develop tolerance to opioids – you might
  need to increase the dose with prolonged use.

- Naloxone 0.4–2 mg IV/SC/IM (maximum 10 mg)
  every 2–3 minutes will reverse the opioid effect, so it
  is useful if respiratory depression or hypotension ensue.
  But, *remember*, the half-life of naloxone is very short,
  so you might have to give repeated doses with long
  half-life opioids (eg, methadone).

- Naloxone is also a good diagnostic tool whenever opioid
  toxicity or abuse is suspected. Naloxone should wake the
  patient up for a few seconds before reverting to his/her
  original state. If respiratory function does not improve
  then question the diagnosis.

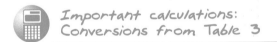

Important calculations: *Conversions from Table 3*

Diamorphine SC injection to oral morphine
30 mg diamorphine daily by syringe driver:
conversion factor = ×3
= 30 × 3
= 90 mg oral morphine OD
= 15 mg oral morphine immediate-release every 4 hours

Morphine IM injection to oral morphine
40 mg morphine daily by injection:
conversion factor = ×2
= 40 × 2
= 80 mg oral morphine OD

Oral morphine to oral tramadol

80 mg oral morphine:

conversion factor = ×0.2

= 80 × 0.2

= 400 mg tramadol total daily dose (ie, 100 mg 6-hourly)

Remember – when converting a patient from regular oral morphine (immediate release) to MST (modified release):

- Add up the total amount of morphine administered in 24 hours (including PRN doses).

- Halve this amount to give an MST BD dose.

- *Example:* 10 mg immediate-release morphine QDS
  = 40 mg in 24 hours
  = 20 mg MST BD

Transdermal fentanyl

The initial fentanyl patch dose should be based on the patient's previous opioid history, including the degree of opioid tolerance, if any. Patches must be replaced every 72 hours. A recommended conversion scheme from oral morphine is given in **Table 4**.

The initial evaluation of the analgesic effect of transdermal fentanyl should not be made before the patch has been worn for 24 hours – there is a gradual increase in serum fentanyl concentration up to this time. Previous analgesic therapy should therefore be phased out gradually from the time of the first application of the patch until analgesic efficacy with fentanyl is attained. Additional breakthrough doses of analgesia might still be required on continuation of the patch.

Remember – fentanyl levels fall gradually once the patch is removed. It can take up to 17 hours for the fentanyl serum concentration to decrease by 50%.

Table 4. Recommended starting doses of transdermal fentanyl if converting from oral morphine.

Oral 24-hour morphine (mg/day)	Transdermal fentanyl dose[a] (µg/hour)
<135	25
135–224	50
225–314	75
315–404	100
405–494	125
495–584	150
585–674	175
675–764	200
765–854	225
855–944	250
945–1,034	275
1,035–1,124	300
[a]Refer to product monograph and seek specialist advice.	

2 Patient-controlled Analgesia

Suparna Bali

What is patient-controlled analgesia?

Patient-controlled analgesia is used for the control of moderate to severe pain in the acute post-operative period. It allows patients to self-administer small, pre-programmed boluses of IV or SC opioids at the push of a button. A lock-out time (ie, a set time limit within which additional boluses cannot be delivered) is also programmed, thereby reducing the risk of overdose.

Advantages of this system include:

- fewer adverse effects and faster recovery time

- no repeated IM or SC injections

- avoids the 'peaks and troughs' of opioid levels

- patient empowerment, with improved individualisation of drug doses resulting in a reduced level of anxiety

- less nursing time

Remember – running a simultaneous background opioid infusion can prevent a post-operative patient from waking up in pain. Consult your anaesthetist if you think this is appropriate.

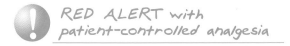

RED ALERT with patient-controlled analgesia

Always check the patient's suitability.
Contraindications include:

- a patient who can't understand the concept of patient-controlled analgesia (eg, confused, drowsy)

- reduced dexterity (eg, arthritis, burns)

- where opioids are contraindicated

- untrained medical/nursing staff

TOP TIPS in ensuring maximum patient benefit

It is paramount that you educate the patient (preferably pre-operatively) about patient-controlled analgesia.

- Tell the patient how the machine works.

- Reassure them that there is minimal risk of opioid addiction or overdose.

- Explain that they must 'keep pain away' by pressing the button before the pain becomes severe (see **Chapter 1** of this section).

A prescription should include the:

- total amount of drug required

- amount of diluent required

- final drug concentration

- bolus dose

- lock-out period

Plus details of any continuous background infusion that might be required.

Remember – the patient usually comes back from theatre with patient-controlled analgesia already prescribed by the anaesthetist on a special proforma. Always double check!

Epidural Analgesia 3

Suparna Bali

Epidural analgesia is safe and effective in providing pain relief before, during and after a surgical procedure (eg, thoracic, abdominal, obstetric or hip surgery) or in the management of chronic pain. In general, small quantities of local anaesthetic and opioid analgesic agents are used in combination, and are administered by slow infusion into the epidural space. Doses (and therefore side effects) are far less than would be required with systemic administration. Because of this, epidurals can reduce the likelihood of complications such as chest infection, DVT and pressure sores.

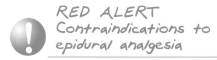

RED ALERT
Contraindications to epidural analgesia

Contraindications include:

- bleeding disorder (including concurrent anti-coagulant therapy; caution with NSAIDs)

- infection/bacteraemia (risk of epidural abscess)

- active local infection of the skin around the epidural site

- hypovolaemia or hypotension

- increased ICP

- allergy to drug(s) used

- spinal disorder (a relative contraindication)

- patient refusal

Choice of opioid

Diamorphine and fentanyl are common options in epidurals: their high lipid solubility means that they pass through the cerebrospinal fluid quickly and therefore have a rapid mode of action. They are also less likely to cause central respiratory depression as they are easily absorbed by local nerve tissue.

Choice of local anaesthetic

Depending on the strength of the local anaesthetic and the size of the nerve, a local anaesthetic can cause a reversible block to nerve conduction. The stronger the local anaesthetic used in epidurals, the more likely it is to block motor as well as sensory function. Weak solutions (eg, 0.125% bupivacaine) can provide good analgesia with minimal or no paraesthesia/paralysis.

Complications in epidural analgesia

Patients might return from theatre with an epidural already *in situ* and prescribed on a special proforma. Your job is to look out for complications and alert the anaesthetist accordingly. These are rare, but it is important that you are aware of them. Here are some examples...

Hypotension and bradycardia
These can result from sympathetic blockade by the local anaesthetic. Once haemorrhage, fluid depletion and an inappropriately high epidural block have been excluded, treat with ephedrine.

Catheter migration
The epidural catheter can migrate from the epidural space to the subarachnoid space, where the opioid is more potent than spinal requirements. This can lead to increased analgesia, sedation and respiratory depression.

Dural puncture headache

If this occurs, lie the patient flat and ensure adequate analgesia and hydration. The patient must avoid straining (eg, treat constipation).

Epidural haematoma

Unintentional placement of the epidural catheter into an epidural blood vessel can cause bleeding into the epidural space, resulting in pressure on the spinal cord. Always routinely check the patient's motor and sensory functions.

Local anaesthetic toxicity

One of the initial symptoms of this is a 'tingling' sensation around the mouth. If not identified quickly, this can lead to more serious consequences including convulsions, coma and cardiac arrest.

Epidural abscess

Infection can occur at the site of the epidural placement and develop into an abscess. Prolonged catheterisation increases the risk.

 TOP TIPS for prescribing epidurals

- Most hospitals have a separate epidural chart (check first), which should include the maximum and minimum rate for the infusion.

- The patient's drug chart must clearly indicate that the patient is receiving an epidural infusion.

- Avoid prescribing other opioid drugs concurrently.

- Pre-empt the side effects associated with opioids and local anaesthetics by prescribing anti-emetics, laxatives and/or anti-histamines.

- Check your hospital guidelines for the INR range within which the epidural catheter can be removed (usually 1–1.5).

Prescribing in Palliative Care

Simon Noble and Clare Turner

(See also **Chapter 1** of this section.)

There is no second chance to improve the quality of life of a dying patient. Getting it right allows a good death and helps lead to an uncomplicated bereavement for the family. However, there is much more to palliative care than whacking up a syringe driver. Liaise early with your palliative care team.

 TOP TIPS for opioid use in palliation

All of the general principles of opioid use apply here (see **Chapter 1** of this section). In addition:

- Don't forget to prescribe an anti-emetic to prevent opioid-induced nausea (haloperidol can help in this regard, although it is generally not thought of as anti-emetic!).

- Always, ALWAYS, *ALWAYS* prescribe a laxative to prevent opioid-induced constipation. The patient will need a softener and a pusher (eg, senna/magnesium hydroxide) (see **Section 3, Chapter 2**).

- Profound constipation secondary to high doses of opioid will probably need something more potent (eg, sodium docusate 100 mg PO TDS).

- Do not prescribe a fentanyl patch first-line for someone with unstable cancer pain: its pharmacokinetics do not allow titration to acute pain.

Is the patient opioid toxic?

Why is it that when a patient has a sodium level of 120 mmol/L, brain metastases and a urinary tract infection, doctors *still* blame the confusion on the morphine?! Think of opioids, sure – but don't become blinded by the opioid light!

Features of opioid toxicity include:

- pin-point pupils

- myoclonus/metabolic flap (like the liver flap)

- drowsiness (severe toxicity)

- respiratory depression (severe toxicity)

- classic visual hallucinations

With the last, patients tend to see dark spots in the periphery of their vision. Many people think they have seen cats, dogs or rats run under the bed. You have to *specifically ask* about this – it is rarely volunteered for fear of being labelled crazy!

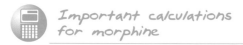

Important calculations for morphine

Breakthrough dose of morphine

Total dose of morphine in 24 hours divided by 6.
Example: a patient is on MST 60 mg BD, so the 24-hour dose is 60 mg × 2 = 120 mg.
Breakthrough dose = 120 mg ÷ 6
= 20 mg PRN

Converting oral morphine to SC diamorphine via the syringe driver

SC diamorphine is three times as potent as oral morphine, so take the 24-hour dose of morphine and divide it by 3.

Example: a patient is on MST 60 mg BD so, as above, the 24-hour dose is 120 mg.
SC diamorphine dose = 120 mg ÷ 3
= 40 mg over 24 hours

Anti-emetics and palliation

(See also **Section 3**.)

Again, all the general principles of nausea and vomiting treatment apply here. Some specifics to palliative care are:

- You might well be using more granisetron or ondansetron as patients will be receiving palliative chemotherapy.

- The degree of nausea or vomiting might be more profound due to toxic drug doses, toxic drugs or disease. Another weapon available to you is levomepromazine (aka Nozinan®), the 'Domestos' of all anti-emetics. Give 12.5–50 mg PO every 4–8 hours, or 12.5–25 mg IV 6- to 8-hourly or SC via a syringe driver. Levomepromazine is not regularly used because it's sedating. Talk to the palliative care team before prescribing it.

Syringe drivers

Syringe drivers are not just for dying patients. There are several important indications for them:

- The patient is unable to swallow or too unwell to take medicines PO.

- The patient is nauseous.

- The patient has poor absorption (eg, bowel stasis, pancreatic dysfunction, hypoalbuminaemia).

Note that, in the palliative care setting, syringe drivers are given SC.

Syringe drivers can be used for the control of pain, nausea, restlessness and colic, amongst other things. When combinations are used, it is important to ensure that the drugs mixed are compatible and do not crystallise. The following commonly used drugs can be mixed together in a syringe driver:

- diamorphine

- haloperidol

- hyoscine hydrobromide

- midazolam

- levomepromazine

- metoclopramide

- cyclizine (maximum concentration, cyclizine 10 mg/mL with diamorphine 50 mg/mL; it can crystallise in saline so use water for injection)

It is unusual to mix more than three drugs together. If you need to use more than three, you should be chatting to the palliative care team or setting up a separate driver.

A useful website for checking drug compatibilities in syringe drivers is www.pallmed.net. Alternatively, refer to an IV injectables guide that gives you the concentrations that the drugs are available in and their compatibilities.

Care in the last 48 hours of life

Once the team has recognised that a patient is dying, the following should be done:

- Stop all unnecessary medicines.

- Ensure that you write-up PRN medicines for all symptomatic eventualities:

  – pain: diamorphine SC PRN

  – agitation: midazolam SC PRN

  – death rattle: hyoscine hydrobromide SC PRN

  – nausea: cyclizine SC PRN

- If the patient is on regular analgesics/anti-emetics, convert to a syringe driver.

- Communicate regularly with the patient's family.

5

Fit for a Fit: Adults with Seizures

Evelyn Frank

What do I do if my patient is fitting? When should I intervene?

In general, don't treat the first fit. If a seizure lasts for more than a few minutes, or if the fits are frequent or occurring without full recovery in between ('status epilepticus'), then it's time to crack on with treatment.

Remember, though, that you do need a good history.

*   Is the patient a known epileptic?

*   Is he/she taking anti-epileptic medication?

*   What is the seizure frequency and how long do they normally last?

*   Is the patient diabetic, pregnant, a known alcoholic or all of the above?

*   Are there likely to be precipitants? Fit thresholds can be lowered by drugs (eg, haloperidol) or infection; some drugs (in toxicity) cause fits; illness (or surgery!) might have prevented the patient from taking their normal medicine; or other drugs might have increased the metabolism or altered the binding of their usual anti-convulsants.

Make sure that you send blood for further investigations (ie, U&Es, LFTs, FBC, glucose, anti-convulsant levels) once you have IV access. Despite all of this, however, seizure treatment is pretty much standardised.

Table 5. Benzodiazepines in the treatment of adult seizures.

Drug	Dose	Top tip
Lorazepam	4 mg IV slow bolus into a large vein, given over 3–5 minutes	Rapid administration increases the risk of respiratory depression and hypotension Lorazepam injection is stored in the fridge
Diazepam emulsion	10 mg IV bolus, maximum 5 mg/minute	Dose can be repeated after 10 minutes
Diazepam	0.5 mg/kg (usually up to 30 mg) PR	Use a half-dose in the elderly Diazepam rectal tubes are available
Midazolam	10 mg buccal	Draw up 10 mg/2 mL and squirt onto the buccal mucosa in the mouth Unlicensed use

Early stage

Benzodiazepines

If IV access is available, and you have full 'resus' equipment available, give IV lorazepam (this is best, as it's shorter acting and has limited tissue loading) or diazepam (see **Table 5**). If no IV access is possible or if you are alone, without support and 'resus', rectal diazepam or buccal midazolam are alternatives.

If the seizure has not been aborted after about 20 minutes, there is incomplete recovery between fits, there is marked hypoxia associated with the fits or there are other worrying factors (eg, haemodynamic compromise, suspected associated head or neck injury), *call an anaesthetist or ICU staff to help* – and roll up your sleeves and get ready for the next step!

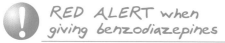

RED ALERT when giving benzodiazepines

- Carefully monitor respiratory rate and blood pressure, especially when administering IV.

- Do not give IM (slow absorption).

- Diazepam injections cause thrombophlebitis – always use Diazemuls®.

- Take special care in the elderly and reduce the dose.

Established status epilepticus

First-line

Your first-line drug is *phenytoin*.

TOP TIPS for phenytoin administration

- Dose: 15 mg/kg – a standard 1 g loading dose is suitable for most patients, but you should calculate the dose for very tiny and very large patients.

- Maximum rate 50 mg/minute – a 1 g loading dose must be given over a minimum of 20 minutes (give undiluted via a syringe driver).

- Alternatively, dilute in 100 mL of 0.9% sodium chloride and infuse over a minimum of 20 minutes using an infusion pump.

- Prescribe a maintenance dose of 300 mg OD, adjusted according to plasma levels (see **Section 7, Chapter 4**).

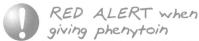

RED ALERT when giving phenytoin

- Always use an inline filter (0.2–0.5 μm) when administering diluted phenytoin.

- Administer via a large vein (phenytoin is very irritant).

- Do not use in patients who are already taking phenytoin unless you know their plasma level.

- ECG monitoring is required for IV loading doses.

- Phenytoin causes further respiratory depression.

- Never give IM.

Second-line

Your second-line drug is *phenobarbitone*.

The ancient drug phenobarbitone is used in patients who can't have phenytoin (eg, a patient who is already on phenytoin and whose blood level is unknown). It is also used in addition to phenytoin if seizures are not controlled despite adequate levels.

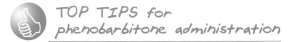

TOP TIPS for phenobarbitone administration

- Loading dose: 10 mg/kg.

- Maximum rate: 60 mg/minute.

- Administration: dilute with 10 times its volume in water for injection immediately before use. Give via a syringe driver.

- Maintenance dose: 60 mg QDS, adjusted according to plasma levels.

And finally...

If, despite all of your valiant efforts, your patient is still fitting then you need the help of an anaesthetist/neurologist/intensivist. By the way, your patient should be on the ICU by now...

Insomnia

6

Jane Ng

If a patient's sleep is disturbed then you will be too. When called, the temptation is to just 'write something up'. But before you do, *stop and think*. Does the patient really need a sedative? Prescribing a hypnotic drug is often undesirable for two reasons:

* Physical and psychological dependence can occur.

* It is difficult to predict the dose needed, and thus the unwanted effects:

  – Patients can feel 'hung-over' or drowsy the next day, reducing their motivation and thus impairing hydration, nutrition and/or mobilisation.

  – If the patient is teetering on the brink of respiratory failure, hypnotics can precipitate it.

  – Benzodiazepines can cause confusion and ataxia in the elderly.

So, don't be bullied into prescribing! First, ask yourself why the patient is not sleeping. What conservative measures can be used? **Table 6** gives some options for non-drug management. Some patients, however, might benefit from a short course of drug intervention – see **Table 7**.

The algorithm in **Figure 1** (p. 134) will help you to choose a drug, while **Table 8** outlines some common doses for insomnia treatment. There are no firm data to distinguish zopiclone (or zaleplon and zolpidem) from other hypnotics, so they should only be used if side effects are experienced with the drugs recommended in the table and figure.

Table 6. Non-drug options in the management of the insomniac patient.

Cause of insomnia	Non-drug response
Noisy environment	Separate from noisy patients
	Move away from ward entrance
	Give foam ear plugs
Lights	Avoid switching the lights on
	Move away from the nurses' station
	If safe, draw curtains around the patient's bed
	Give an eye mask
Cold	More blankets?
Fear – general or specific (eg, "I might die in the night")	Talk to the patient
	Get psychologist help
Hunger	Give food later at night
	Give a nasogastric feed top-up by day
Steroids	Try to avoid evening dosages
Needing to pass urine	Catheter?
	Reduce overnight fluids
	Avoid late use of diuretics
Disrupted day/night cycle	Keep the patient awake all day (ask relatives to come in if needs be), then give peace and quiet (see above!) at a set time
	A clock helps orientation, as does facing a window
Other	Avoid coffee late at night
	Give a hot, milky drink
	Give a 'night cap' if alcohol is not contraindicated

Table 7. Reasons to prescribe drugs.

Reason	Action
Alcohol withdrawal People often understate their alcohol consumption – it is not just the patient with all the signs of chronic liver disease who could be withdrawing!	Prevention is better than cure! See **Section 1, Chapter 8**
Nicotine withdrawal Think of this in all smokers, not just the COPD patient	Nicotine patch
Disrupted day/night cycle	A short course of short-acting sedation at night, in conjunction with the non-pharmacological measures in **Table 6**, can help
Dependence on night sedation If the patient has been on nitrazepam 10 mg at night for 15 years, it's a bit cruel to let them go 'cold turkey'	Give them their usual drug!
Pain	Give appropriate analgesia
Acute confusional state 'Seeing things' can be scary; paranoia can also keep a patient awake	Address all physiological causes Talk to the patient If still unresponsive, drugs might be needed – see **Section 1, Chapter 7**

Table 8. Common doses for insomnia treatment.

Drug	Adult dose (mg)	Dose in the elderly patient (mg)
Nitrazepam	5–10	2.5–5
Diazepam	5–15	2.5–7.5
Temazepam	5–10	2.5–5
Zopiclone	7.5	3.75
Chlorpromazine	10–25	5–12.5
Promazine	Not used in younger adults	25–50
Promethazine	25–50	25–50

Figure 1. Choosing appropriate sedation.

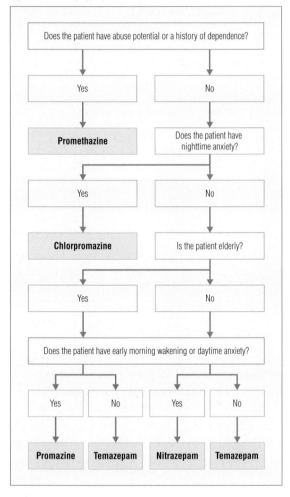

TOP TIPS in prescribing sedation

Try not to! Ensure that you have thought of all possible causes for the insomnia and have treated these first.

If you *do* have to prescribe sedation:

- Prescribe only as stat or PRN, not regular.

- State a review date on the prescription: tolerance can develop within 3–14 days, so it makes no sense to continue in the long-term.

- Avoid prescribing dose ranges, as the higher dose might be given without good cause.

- Use the lowest possible dose of the shortest-acting agents.

- Hypnotics can take 15–60 minutes to take effect, so give them at least 30 minutes before the patient wants to sleep.

Some final thoughts

Remember these final pointers:

- Benzodiazepines are the main culprits for withdrawal (although withdrawal is possible for all of the drugs mentioned). In general, the drug should be slowly tapered off after 2 weeks of regular use. A possible regimen is given in **Figure 2**.

- Always be aware of withdrawal symptoms – they can occur with <2 weeks of regular therapy.

- Try not to discharge patients on hypnotics.

- If there is an underlying psychiatric condition, discuss the problem with a psychiatrist – anti-psychotics, anti-depressants or other anxiolytics might be indicated. *Beware* – hypnotics can worsen depressive states and interact with the aforementioned classes of drugs.

Figure 2. A possible regimen for tapering off benzodiazepines.

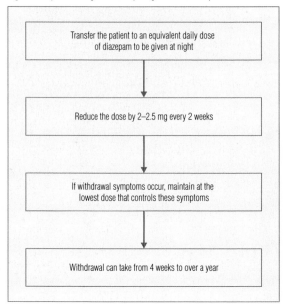

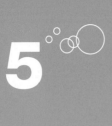

5

Blood

1. Warfarin Prescribing   139

2. Parenteral Anti-coagulation   146

Warfarin Prescribing

Bridget Coleman

Warfarin is highly effective at killing rats. In the hands of the uneducated, it is just as effective at killing humans. So to get it right every time…

Starting treatment with warfarin

Speedy anti-coagulation (eg, DVT, PE, mechanical heart valve)

Days 1 and 2: start warfarin along with heparin/LMWH (see the next chapter). Traditionally, warfarin 10 mg is given on days 1 and 2. However, regimens with lower doses (eg, 8 mg or 5 mg) are increasingly being used.

Day 3: take daily INRs until the patient stabilises and a maintenance dose is established.

Nomograms will guide you through the initial dose adjustments. **Table 1** shows one we made earlier! Whatever your plan, all patients should receive heparin for at least 4 days. Heparin should not be discontinued until the INR stays within the therapeutic range for at least 2 days.

Less speedy anti-coagulation (eg, out-patients, AF)

Days 1–5: give warfarin 5 mg OD. In risky situations (see the Red Alert), give 3 mg OD.

Day 6: return for INR – adjust dose in response to INR.

Table 1. Recommended warfarin doses to be used to achieve the desired INR after loading.

Day	INR	Dose (mg)
3	<1.5	5–10
	1.5–1.9	2.5–5
	2–3	0–5
	>3	0
4	<1.5	10
	1.5–1.9	5–7.5
	2–3	0–5
	>3	0
5	<1.5	10
	1.5–1.9	7.5–10
	2–3	0–5
	>3	0
6	<1.5	7.5–12.5
	1.5–1.9	5–10
	2–3	0–7.5
	>3	0

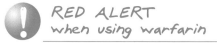

RED ALERT
when using warfarin

- Take a baseline INR before treatment.

- Very high INRs can be produced in sensitive patients.

- Patients with protein C and protein S deficiency risk warfarin-induced skin necrosis if anti-coagulation is excessive (areas of fat, eg, breast, buttock, thigh).

- *Beware* in certain disease states (eg, congestive cardiac failure, liver impairment)!

- *Beware* of drug interactions (see p. 142)!

Table 2. Target INRs for various conditions requiring warfarin.

Reason for warfarin therapy	Target INR
AF	2.5
DVT/PE	2.5
Recurrence of DVT/PE whilst on warfarin	3.5
Mechanical valve replacement	2.5–3.5 (dependent on position and type of valve)

- *Beware* in the elderly! Older patients need lower doses of warfarin and often have concurrent medical conditions, so they might already be on medications that will interact with warfarin.

Adjusting the dose of warfarin in the longer term

The target depends upon the reason for anti-coagulation. **Table 2** shows these targets.

Adjusting the dose can be more of an art than a science, aiming to get the INR within 0.5 either way of the target. In practice, a short-term deviation by up to ±0.75 units is acceptable (eg, for a target INR of 2.5, anywhere between 1.75 and 3.25 is usually acceptable).

 TOP TIPS in INR targeting

- Don't over-react to individual INRs! Often it is enough to reduce/increase the dose for just 1 or 2 days to allow the INR to get back on target.

- Dose adjustments should be by ±10%. Occasionally, you will need to adjust by ±20%, particularly during the early stages of treatment.

- Booster stat doses should be about 150% of the usual maintenance dose.

- Don't measure the INR too frequently! A single dose doesn't start to have an effect for 12–16 hours and lasts for 4–5 days. So unless you have particular concerns, it is pointless to measure the INR more than twice a week during hospital admission.

- The anti-coagulant clinic is a good source of advice. Pick up that phone!

- Again, *beware* in the elderly – they need closer monitoring.

Anti-coagulation in the elderly

The elderly generally:

- need lower doses of warfarin

- have a greater number of other medical conditions and concurrent drug use, which can affect INR stability or alter the risk of bleeding

Consequently, older people need to be monitored more carefully.

Reversing the effects of warfarin

Before you reach for the vitamin K, stop! Does the patient really need it? Vitamin K certainly will work within 6 hours and will bring the INR into therapeutic range in 24 hours. However, it can also make the patient resistant to warfarin for days, maybe even weeks, especially at doses >2 mg. IV vitamin K is rarely indicated, except where there is life-threatening bleeding. **Table 3** has a good plan to follow.

Drug–drug interactions

Drugs can affect the INR in warfarinised patients by:

Table 3. Recommended interventions where the INR is elevated.

Event	Action
Life-threatening bleeding	Stop warfarin
	Give vitamin K 5 mg PO/IV
	Give FFP for 'immediate' effect
INR >8	Stop warfarin
	If there are other risk factors for bleeding, give vitamin K 0.5–2.5 mg PO
INR 6–8	Stop warfarin for 1–2 days
INR 3.5–6 (target 2.5)	Reduce dose or stop warfarin for 1–2 days
INR 4–6 (target 3.5)	Reduce dose or stop warfarin for 1–2 days

- altering drug binding, or…

- …altering drug metabolism

But remember, drugs that affect vitamin K absorption (eg, those causing/treating malabsorption or altering bowel flora) will also make a huge difference. It is therefore best to treat *any* drug as having the potential to interact with warfarin. However, in practice, the drugs in **Table 4** tend to cause most of the difficulties seen.

Drug–food interactions

Who said greens were good for you? Patients taking health foods, food supplements and exceptionally large quantities of green vegetables (which contain a lot of vitamin K) have seen their INR take a skydive. Problem foods include turnips, greens, beetroot, broccoli, cabbage, lettuce and spinach. Healthy portions, however, are fine.

An example: anti-coagulant clinic staff were at a loss to explain why one man's INR was dropping like a stone… until he owned up to being on the cabbage soup diet!

Table 4. Drugs associated with warfarin interactions.

Drug	Action
Amiodarone	Increases INR in most patients
	Onset is slow, but usually develops within 2 weeks. Monitor the patient on a weekly basis for the first 4 weeks of treatment
	Interactions can persist for many weeks after the amiodarone has been withdrawn
Antibiotics	Highly unpredictable: broad-spectrum antibiotics often raise INR, but rarely reduce it
	In practice, a slight decrease in warfarin dose (eg, 0.5 mg) for the duration of the course might be advisable
Alcohol	Binge drinking dramatically increases INR
	Chronic heavy alcohol usage can increase warfarin requirements
Aspirin	Not good news! Analgesic doses of aspirin increase the chance of bleeding, damage the stomach wall and can increase the INR. Triple whammy!
	Low-dose aspirin (75–150 mg) appears to be safer, and in some circumstances is co-prescribed with warfarin
NSAIDs	As for aspirin
	Avoid if possible. If absolutely necessary then ibuprofen/diclofenac are considered the safest options, but use the lowest effective dose and monitor closely

Drug–disease interactions

Changes in a patient's clinical condition can interfere with warfarin control. The effect of warfarin is enhanced with:

- liver impairment

- exacerbation of congestive cardiac failure

- renal impairment

- infective episodes

- steatorrhoea

And reduced with:

- diarrhoea

- vomiting

Liaising with the anti-coagulant clinic

The anti-coagulant clinic needs a great deal of information to be able to manage a patient properly. Local referral forms are usually available, but the minimum information they need is likely to be:

- diagnosis

- target INR and duration of therapy

- last three INR values and warfarin doses

- other drugs taken

- any risk factors for bleeding

Most clinics will not accept a patient unless they have all of the relevant details. Check what your clinic needs and save yourself some phone calls!

2 Parenteral Anti-coagulation

Rob Shulman

Successful anti-coagulation requires a fine balance between clotting and bleeding, which can easily go wrong. The good news is that even the thickest clot can manage coagulation, if they apply some simple principles!

There are two forms of heparin available: LMWH SC and unfractionated heparin IV (occasionally SC).

Low molecular weight heparins

LMWHs are simpler and more convenient to use than unfractionated heparin. There are several agents on the market, but the main ones are enoxaparin (Clexane®) and dalteparin (Fragmin®).

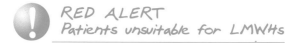

RED ALERT
Patients unsuitable for LMWHs

Do not use treatment-dose LMWHs in:

*   the severely obese

*   paediatric patients (unless under specialist advice)

*   those in whom you might need to stop the anti-coagulation suddenly (eg, at risk of a bleed or need to go for surgery at an unpredicted time)

*   those with moderate/severe renal impairment (creatinine clearance <30 mL/minute)

Table 5. Recommended LMWH doses for the management of DVTs and PEs.

Use	Drug and dose
Treatment of DVT/PE	Enoxaparin 1.5 mg/kg SC OD or dalteparin 200 units/kg SC OD (max. 18,000 units/day)
Treatment of DVT with increased likelihood of bleeding	Enoxaparin 1.5 mg/kg SC OD or dalteparin 100 units/kg SC BD

Note: Your hospital might use standard doses specific to a weight band. Check local practices.

For proven DVT/PE, concomitantly commence warfarin as described in the previous chapter. Continue heparin for at least 4 days, and do not stop until the INR has been in the target range for at least 2 days.

Monitoring	
FBC before therapy, and repeat every 72 hours thereafter	Checking for heparin-induced thrombocytopenia APTT ratio and anti-Xa levels are not usually required

Reversal	
Severe	Protamine sulphate 40 mg IV
	Give protamine sulphate IV slowly (5 mg/minute), not more than 50 mg at any one time

Note: LMWH might not be fully reversed by protamine.
Protamine is short-acting, so you might need further doses.

Treatment guidelines for DVT and PE

The recommended LMWH doses are in shown in **Table 5**.

IV unfractionated heparin

For the management of massive PE, see **Section 2, Chapter 7**.

Your pre-infusion standard bloods should be FBC, APTT and prothrombin time.

A loading dose followed by continuous infusion of the unfractionated heparin is often required (see **Table 6**). The infusion rate is dependent upon the APTT ratio (see **Table 7**).

Table 6. Recommended loading doses and infusions of unfractionated heparin.

	Recommendation
Loading dose	For DVT, give an IV bolus of heparin sodium 5,000 units (if <50 kg, use 70–100 units/kg) over 5 minutes
	For PE, give an IV bolus of 80 units/kg (rounded to the nearest 1,000 units) over 5 minutes
Initial infusion rate	Make up 24,000 units of heparin sodium to a final volume of 48 mL with sodium chloride 0.9% injection (final concentration of 500 units/mL)
	Infuse IV initially at 1,000–2,000 units/hour (15–25 units/kg/hour for DVT/PE; usually 20 units/kg/hour)
	Check the APTT ratio after 4–6 hours of starting the infusion (6 hours is better to reflect steady state)
	Adjust the dose in accordance with **Table 7**

Prevention of DVT

All hospitalised patients are at risk of DVT (see **Table 8**), and this risk should be minimised for every patient. LMWHs form the bedrock of prevention.

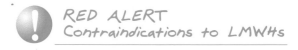

RED ALERT
Contraindications to LMWHs

Contraindications to LMWHs include:

- INR >1.3, APTT ratio >1.3 or platelets <75 × 10⁹/L – consider TED stockings

- Creatinine clearance <30 mL/minute – use half the normal dose of LMWH, or heparin calcium or sodium 5,000 units SC BD

- In neurosurgery patients, *do not* commence anti-coagulation before discussing with the registrar or consultant!

Table 7. Changes in the unfractionated heparin infusion rate required in response to an abnormal APTT ratio.

APTT ratio	Infusion rate change (note: do not use this for heparin infusion post-acute MI)
>7	Stop for 1 hour, recheck APTT ratio and then reduce by 500 units/hour
5.1–7	Reduce by 500 units/hour
4.1–5	Reduce by 300 units/hour
3.1–4	Reduce by 100 units/hour
2.6–3	Reduce by 50 units/hour
1.5–2.5	No change
1.2–1.4	Increase by 200 units/hour
<1.2	Consider 2,500 units IV bolus, increase by 400 units/hour

Monitoring
Daily monitoring of the APTT ratio is essential
The target range for the APTT ratio is between 1.5 and 2.5 times the control. Target ranges can differ between laboratories so make sure that you check yours!
After each dose change, wait 4–6 hours before taking blood for the next APTT ratio (6 hours is better to reflect steady state)
Assays should be taken more frequently (eg, 4-hourly) if the APTT ratio is >5
Repeat FBC every 72 hours in case heparin-induced thrombocytopenia develops

Reversal	
In severe bleeding	Protamine sulphate 1 mg IV for every 100 units of heparin given over the previous hour
	Halve the protamine dose if the heparin infusion has been stopped for 1 hour, quarter the dose if it has been stopped for 2 hours

Notes:

Heparin has a short half-life, so stopping the infusion is usually enough.

If protamine sulphate is required, give it IV slowly (5 mg/minute), not more than 50 mg at a time.

Protamine is short-acting, so you might need further doses.

The APTT ratio can be checked as early as 5–15 minutes after a protamine dose.

Even if the APTT ratio is initially corrected, recheck at 2 hours and again at 5–8 hours after protamine administration – there is a possibility of heparin rebound.

Consult a haematologist for advice.

Table 8. DVT risks in different patient groups.

Risk category	Definition	Therapy
Medical patients		
High	All hospitalised medical patients aged >40 years	LMWH OD (eg, enoxaparin 40 mg or dalteparin 5,000 units SC OD) until patient mobilises (except for head-injury patients and those in the excluded groups mentioned in the Red Alert on p. 148)
		The role of heparin or warfarin in acute stroke remains unclear
Orthopaedic surgery		
High	Elective hip or knee replacement Hip fracture or major limb fracture	LMWH OD (eg, enoxaparin 40 mg or dalteparin 5,000 units SC OD) until patient mobilises Your unit might prefer to use lower doses to avoid bleeding. An alternative is intermittent compression boots
General surgery		
High	Major general surgery, aged >60 years Major general surgery, aged 40–60 years, and cancer or history of DVT/PE Thrombophilia (patients with a proven specific haemostatic defect)	LMWH OD (eg, enoxaparin 40 mg or dalteparin 5,000 units SC OD) until patient mobilises Consider TED stockings
Moderate	Major general surgery, aged 40–60 years, without other risk factors Minor surgery, aged >60 years Minor surgery, aged 40–60 years, with history of DVT/PE or on oestrogen therapy	LMWH OD (eg, enoxaparin 20 mg SC OD or dalteparin 2,500 units SC daily) Early mobilisation

Table 8. *Continued.*

Risk category	Definition	Therapy
Low	Major general surgery, aged <40 years, without other risk factors	Early mobilisation
	Minor surgery, aged 40–60 years, without other risk factors	

Risk factors: the risk is increased by infectious disease, the presence of varicose veins, general immobility, obesity, oestrogen-containing oral contraceptives and hormone replacement therapy.

Minor surgery: operations, other than abdominal, lasting <45 minutes.

Major surgery: any intra-abdominal operation and all other operations lasting >45 minutes.

Note: there is an ongoing risk of DVT in high-risk surgical patients for up to 5 weeks post-operation.

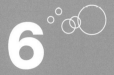

6

Surgery

1. Practical Prescribing in
   the Surgical Patient   155

2. Diabetes and Surgery   163

3. Bowel Preparation   166

Practical Prescribing in the Surgical Patient

Rebecca White

The issues surrounding prescribing for the surgical patient can be divided into two:

- Prescribing drugs required as a consequence of the surgery itself (eg, analgesia, anti-emetics, thromboprophylaxis, antibiotics, fluids).

- Managing any medications that the patient was taking prior to their surgery during the metabolically stressful and potentially starved post-operative period.

Most hospitals have policies and protocols relating to peri-operative prescribing. Look yours up and then supplement with the following guide…

Nil by mouth

For elective operations, patients undergoing a general anaesthetic should not take solids orally for 6 hours prior to surgery, to limit the risk of aspiration. However, the more recent trend is to allow clear fluids until 2 hours before surgery. The evidence demonstrates that this improves gastric motility, thereby reducing the aspiration risk further. Therefore, you may give routine medications with clear fluids until 2 hours before surgery.

If no enteral absorption is likely – or where reliable absorption is essential – then a switch to parenteral preparations might be needed. Consult your pharmacist – many doses change as the route changes.

Local anaesthetic procedures do not generally require the patient to be NBM. However, some anaesthetists prefer the patient to be made NBM if there is a chance that a general anaesthetic might be needed. Check with the anaesthetist!

Routine drug modification

Always consider the risk–benefit ratio of continuing or discontinuing a medication.

Anti-coagulation

See also **Section 5, Chapter 2** on anti-coagulation and heparin.

Anti-platelet agents: aspirin, clopidogrel, dipyridamole

These should be discontinued 7 days prior to most major operations, and restarted the day after surgery. For some operations, however, the benefit of continuing the anti-platelet agent outweighs the risk (eg, carotid endarterectomy).

Warfarin

Details depend on the indication for warfarin and the operation being performed.

- For AF, previous DVT or PE: stop warfarin 3–4 days prior to surgery. Commence standard thromboprophylaxis (see **Section 5, Chapter 2**) on admission.

- For heart valves: stop warfarin 3–4 days prior to surgery. Once the INR is <2, commence an unfractionated heparin infusion. Stop this infusion 2 hours prior to surgery.

Whether and when to restart anti-coagulation will depend on the operation being performed. If strict control is required, continue the heparin infusion post-operatively, simultaneously reload on warfarin and stop the heparin infusion when the

Table 1. Steroid cover required prior to surgery.

Steroid dose	Type of surgery	
	Minor	**Major**
Low dose (eg, prednisolone 5 mg/day)	Give usual oral dose prior to surgery Resume usual oral dose post-operatively	Pre-operative: prednisolone 5 mg PO Peri-operative: hydrocortisone 25 mg IV Post-operative: hydrocortisone 25 mg IV 8-hourly for 48 hours, then resume regular oral dose
High dose (eg, prednisolone 40 mg/day)	Give usual oral dose prior to surgery Resume usual oral dose post-operatively	Pre-operative: prednisolone 40 mg PO Peri-operative: hydrocortisone 50 mg IV Post-operative: hydrocortisone 50 mg IV 8-hourly for 72 hours, then resume regular oral dose

INR is therapeutic. However, it might be decided that it is too risky to restart anti-coagulation (eg, following neurosurgery).

Anti-diabetic agents and insulin
See the next chapter.

Steroids
See also **Section 7, Chapter 2**.

Steroid replacement is necessary if the patient is currently on steroids or has received a prolonged course of steroids in the preceding 3 months (see **Table 1**). This is to reduce the risk of hypoadrenal crisis due to the stress response of surgery.

Anti-epileptics, anti-Parkinsonian medication and immunosuppressants
These groups of medicines are usually continued during the peri-operative period as the consequences of discontinuation

could be serious. Most are available in parenteral or rectal formulations, but bioavailability differs and expert advice should always be sought before changing the route of administration – ideally *before* the patient goes to theatre!

Requirements following surgery
Fluids
How much of what?

- Examine the patient (revise the signs of a dry and over-loaded patient) and read their chart. Estimate how much fluid they are 'down' from theatre and how 'dry' they are, and aim to make this up at an appropriate rate – if hypotensive and compromised, *now!* If slightly dry, over a few hours.

- Then add the 'normal' rate of requirement (25–50 mL/kg/day allows for urinary, faecal and insensible losses)…

- … and then add 'extra' losses (eg, sweat, diarrhoea, stoma).

- Estimate what the patient is losing. Salt? Bicarbonate? Water? Potassium?

- Consider deficiencies – are they already low in K⁺? Do they need blood or clotting products?

- Consider the rate needed and how much is safe (eg, you should be more cautious in a patient with known poor cardiac function).

- Now write up an appropriate regimen!

You're not done yet! Make sure that you assess fluid requirements twice daily (more frequently in the sick).

Example
For a routine, 24-hour maintenance fluid regimen in a euvolaemic patient:

- 1 L 0.9% saline, 2 L 5% dextrose and 20 mmol K⁺ with each dextrose bag, or...

- ...3 L Hartmann's solution

Note: there is growing evidence that balanced electrolyte solutions – such as Ringer's lactate and Hartmann's solution – make better fluids than so-called 'normal saline'.

Analgesia

See also **Section 4, Chapter 1**.

Revise the analgesic ladder (see p. 105) – post-operative pain control employs the 'step-down' approach. All patients should be on regular paracetamol and/or NSAIDs. In addition, many will need an opioid. Gradually move down the ladder until the patient is off all analgesia. Commonly used analgesics and their doses are given in **Section 4, Table 1**.

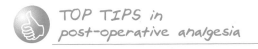

TOP TIPS *in*
post-operative analgesia

Regular simple analgesia should be the baseline – there is never a place for morphine in the absence of regular paracetamol (PO, PR or IV). This reduces opioid doses and thus side effects.

- When clinically indicated, a regular NSAID can be added to paracetamol – again sparing opioid doses. Beware renal risks (see **Section 1, Chapter 5**).

- Regular opioid use will usually cause constipation. *Always* prescribe a stimulant laxative such as senna *at the same time* – don't wait until the patient is constipated as obstruction can result and straining at stool isn't the best approach for an abdominal wound! Lactulose is ineffective for this indication.

- Codeine is weakly effective in approximately 30% of patients and totally ineffective (due to the genetics of the patient) in 5–10%. It is therefore unreliable! Codeine is metabolised to morphine anyway, so why not cut out the middle man and prescribe morphine from the start?

- Tramadol often causes severe dysphoria and hallucinations, especially in older patients. The best advice, then, is to stick to morphine/fentanyl, paracetamol and NSAIDs as your baseline!

Post-operative nausea and vomiting

Use a 'step-up' approach: start with one drug, then add a second (and then a third) from a different class. For example:

- cyclizine: 50 mg PO/IV/IM TDS

- prochlorperazine: 10 mg PO TDS, 12.5 mg IM (followed in 6 hours by an oral dose), 25 mg PR (followed in 6 hours by an oral dose)

- granisetron: 1 mg PO/IV/SC BD

 TOP TIPS in post-operative nausea and vomiting

- Domperidone and metoclopramide are not particularly effective for this indication and are inadvisable immediately following GI surgery.

- Always consider *why* the patient is vomiting. Can you reduce their opioids? Are they obstructed? Do they have an ileus?

- Once you have identified the problem, give anti-emetics regularly rather than intermittently. Vomiting is horrid and misery-making and, with an abdominal wound, it hurts like hell and can prevent healing. On top of all that, it also upsets the patient's fluid and electrolyte balance.

Prophylaxis

Thromboprophylaxis

See **Section 5, Chapter 2**.

Antibiotic prophylaxis

Antibiotic prescribing is usually protocol driven. Most patients require only one pre-operative dose. Therapy continued post-operatively is only of benefit in proven infections.

Patients with cardiac valve lesions/artificial valves will require extra antibiotic cover (see **Section 7, Chapter 3**).

Splenectomy prophylaxis

1. Prescribe (2 weeks prior to elective splenectomy or 2 weeks after emergency splenectomy):

   - pneumococcal vaccine 0.5 mL IM

   - *Hemophilus influenzae* type B vaccine 0.5 mL IM

   - meningococcal conjugated C vaccine 0.5 mL IM

2. Prescribe lifelong penicillin V 250–500 mg PO BD (or erythromycin 250–500 mg BD if allergic to penicillin).

3. Give the patient a splenectomy card to take away.

High-output stomas

Jejunostomies

These usually require specialist input. Treatment options include:

- dietetics input for a low-residue, high-salt diet

- high-dose loperamide 4–8 mg QDS and/or codeine 60–120 mg QDS

- addition of a PPI

- oral fluid restriction and hypertonic salt solutions PO

- replacement of sodium, magnesium and calcium PRN IV

- octreotide (but only as a last resort if all the above measures have failed!)

Ileostomies

If you can find no identifiable cause, prescribe loperamide 2–4 mg PO or codeine 60 mg PO before meals. Involve dietetics and stoma specialists.

Colostomies

You should rule out causes other than surgery (eg, antibiotics, obstruction, overflow). Use loperamide with caution. Get advice from dietetics and stoma specialists.

Diabetes and Surgery

Preet Panesar

2

Admission for surgery often involves a period of no calorie intake, so the patient can be at risk of both low and high blood sugars. Together with the metabolic stress of surgery, this can increase insulin resistance and thus push blood sugar up. Poor management in such circumstances can lead to hyperglycaemia, ketoacidosis and post-operative complications.

Pre-operative principles

- Pre-warn the anaesthetist that the patient is a diabetic.

- Ensure that the patient is *first* on the *morning* list.

- Admit patients with type I diabetes at least a day before surgery.

- Admit patients with poorly controlled diabetes, especially those who are in for major surgery, 2–3 days before surgery.

- Ensure that blood sugar levels are monitored at least every 2 hours.

- Aim to keep blood sugar levels between 6 and 12 mmol/L. Regimens for this are given in **Tables 2** and **3**.

Table 2. The pre-operative management of the diabetic patient.

Type of diabetes	Comment
Diet controlled	No specific intervention required
	Monitor blood glucose levels
Type 2, tablet controlled	Stop short-acting sulphonylureas (eg, gliclazide) on the morning of surgery
	Stop long-acting sulphonylureas (eg, glibenclamide) 2–3 days prior to surgery. Convert to a short-acting sulphonylurea or insulin if needed
	Stop metformin 48 hours prior to surgery. Do not restart until at least 48 hours post-operation, or later if renal function has declined. This is to avoid lactic acidosis
	If poor control or major surgery, start an IV insulin infusion
Type 1 and type 2, on insulin	Give the usual SC insulin dose the night before surgery
	Commence NBM period from midnight
	Omit the usual morning dose of insulin
	Convert the usual SC insulin to an IV infusion
	Monitor blood glucose levels and change the infusion rate as appropriate
	IV insulin should be continued until the patient is able to eat and drink. The patient should be given their usual SC dose of insulin, and the IV insulin infusion should be stopped 30 minutes later

Table 3. Interventions required for the diabetic patient undergoing surgery.

Type of diabetes	Type of surgery			
	Minor	Moderate	Major	Emergency
Insulin dependent	Fast and check	Insulin sliding scale or GIK	Insulin sliding scale or GIK	Insulin sliding scale
Non-insulin dependent	Fast and check	Fast and check	Insulin sliding scale or GIK	Insulin sliding scale

Post-operative therapy

- Continue to monitor blood glucose levels and electrolytes frequently.

- Ideally, convert back to oral or SC insulin therapy with breakfast as soon as the patient can reliably tolerate an oral diet.

- *Do not* start metformin for 48 hours post-operatively or if renal function has deteriorated.

- For patients who were on insulin pre-operatively, give their usual SC dose of insulin and stop the IV insulin infusion 30 minutes later.

Check your local hospital protocol for insulin sliding scale or GIK regimens (see **Section 1, Chapter 6**).

Remember: poor control can lead to morbidity, delayed discharge and even death!

3 Bowel Preparation

Simon Keady and Olivia Hameer

The type of bowel preparation is dependent upon the time
and type of treatment/investigation. Remember si*C*kly –
*C*heck with local preferences before prescribing, as ineffective
treatments will result in delays and missed theatre slots.

General advice

- Omit solids for at least 8 hours prior to the operation.

- Allow clear fluids only during this time.

- Available preparations include those shown in **Table 4**.

Table 4. Bowel cleansing regimens used prior to investigations.

Laxative	Typical dose	Additional information
Klean-Prep®	4 sachets in 4 L within 4–6 hours of the procedure, or 2 sachets in the evening before the procedure and a further 2 on the morning of the examination	Until 4 L drunk or clear discharge
Citramag®	1 sachet at 8 am the day before the procedure, then 1 sachet 6–8 hours later	Use half this dose for elderly patients
Fleet® Phospho-soda®	45 mL diluted with half a glass of cold water followed by a glass of cold water	–
	If the patient is undergoing a morning procedure, give the first dose at 7 am and the second dose at 7 pm on the day before the procedure	
	If an afternoon procedure, give the first dose at 7 pm on the day before the procedure and the second dose at 7 am on the day of the procedure	
Picolax®	1 sachet at 8 am the day before the procedure then 1 sachet 6–8 hours later	Heat is generated on reconstitution. Will work within 3 hours of the first dose

7

Miscellaneous

1.	Calculations for the Prescriber	171
2.	Corticosteroids	176
3.	Infections	179
4.	Therapeutic Drug Monitoring	192
5.	Drug Hypersensitivities and Contraindications	204
6.	Interactions that Matter	209
7.	Intravenous Therapy	218

Calculations for the Prescriber

1

Simon Keady

From ICU to the paediatric ward, your practical skills of calculation are going to be tested. Days of 'double maths daydreams' will haunt you, especially when you're tired. What you need is a simple, straightforward strategy...

Rule 1. Be clear about your units

Do the maths in two directions, and make sure it works

Take the example of an 85-year-old patient with metastatic bowel cancer to whom you are providing palliative care. He has been asking for a total of 60 mg PRN morphine a day, and the palliative care nurse is recommending an SC morphine infusion.

a. You need to give 60 mg morphine in 24 hours.

b. Morphine comes in various concentrations – one is 30 mg in 1 mL. Therefore, you need two vials of the drug, totalling 2 mL.

c. SC pumps come in various sizes – one is a 30 mL pump. Therefore, you need to prescribe 2 mL of morphine made up to a total of 30 mL with water.

d. Run this pump over 24 hours, ie, the pump will run at a rate of 1.25 mL/hour.

Now, work this backwards:

a. 1.25 mL contains 2.5 mg morphine.

b. 2.5 mg morphine/hour equates to 60 mg morphine in 24 hours.

You've done it right!

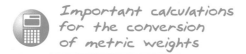

Important calculations for the conversion of metric weights

- 1 kilogram (kg) = 1,000 grams (g)

- 1 gram (g) = 1,000 milligrams (mg)

- 1 milligram (mg) = 1,000 micrograms (µg)

- 1 microgram (µg) = 1,000 nanograms (ng)

- 1 litre (L) = 1,000 millilitres (mL)

Rule 2. Do a 'commonsense check'

How many vials of a drug am I asking a nurse to reconstitute? *That* many? Am I really going to give that 3-year-old a dose I would normally give to an adult? Is that patient really going to need a whole bottle of medicine four times a day?!

Rule 3. Always, ALWAYS, *ALWAYS* get someone to double-check you

When you are most tired, you are most confident – and also most likely to make an error.

Percentages

Percentages can be very confusing! Two key facts help:

Fact 1

A percentage value is a weight or a volume in 100 mL, eg:

- 0.9% (w/v) sodium chloride is 0.9 g per 100 mL

- 5% (w/v) dextrose is 5 g per 100 mL

So 5% dextrose won't help to treat or prevent hypoglycaemia very well – you need more sugar (eg, 10% or 50% dextrose, ie, 10 g/100 mL or 50 g/100 mL).

Fact 2

Diluting will always give you a lower percentage. So for the patient who needs an epidural, starting with 25 mL of 0.25% bupivacaine and diluting down to 50 mL with 0.9% sodium chloride will double the volume and halve the final concentration to 0.125%.

Ratios

Ratios can be just as tricky! But here there's only one key fact…

Key fact

The weight is always in grams and the volume in millilitres.

For instance, adrenaline is commonly available in two strengths:

- adrenaline 1 in 10,000 = 1 g in 10,000 mL = 0.1 mg/mL

- adrenaline 1 in 1,000 = 1 g in 1,000 mL = 1 mg/mL

In the peri-arrest situation, you might want to give 'a bit' of adrenaline. If there's not enough time to draw the exact concentration you want, grab the 1 in 1,000 adrenaline from the crash trolley and dilute it – eg, take out 10 mL from a 100 mL bag of 0.9% sodium chloride and replace it with the 10 mL minijet 1 in 1,000 adrenaline from the crash trolley. Give it a shake. You now have adrenaline at 0.1 mg in 1 mL.

Gravity flow administration

Gravity flow administration sets all have a specific number of drops/mL by which they administer infusion fluids. Nursing staff are an invaluable source of information in ensuring that what you want to prescribe can be easily administered.

Once you have worked out at how many mL/hour you want to run your drug, you can work out how many drops/minute are needed, and you can estimate if you have fixed the administration set correctly.

The exception: take care for all of your cardiac patients who need amiodarone – the drop size is reduced through gravity flow sets. *Always* use a pump.

 TOP TIPS for gravity flow administration sets (adult systems)

- Standard administration set: 20 drops/mL.

- Blood administration set: 15 drops/mL.

- Burette administration: 60 drops/mL.

Infusion administration

Other infusions are delivered through medical devices (usually a volumetric pump or syringe driver), which deliver a volume as mL/hour. The majority of these devices require syringes to be made to a final volume of 50 mL.

Not all drugs are administered at the same concentration and you need to recognise this at an early stage. For example, morphine is administered as a dose/hour, while drugs such as dopamine and dobutamine are administered as a dose/minute. Failure to get these the right way round will have serious consequences!

So, go back to siCkly, and Check, CHECK, *CHECK* your calculations and prescription!

2 Corticosteroids

Rob Shulman

Converting from one steroid to another is often necessary and can cause much head scratching. But help is at hand with **Table 1**! As an example, hydrocortisone 50 mg IV QDS can be converted to prednisolone 50 mg PO OM.

Management of steroid therapy

To maximise the benefit and minimise the risk of corticosteroid therapy, think of the following:

- Use the lowest possible dose for the shortest length of time.

- Steroid tablets given in the morning and on alternate days can reduce adrenal suppression.

- Nighttime doses can cause insomnia, so try not to prescribe a dose after 6 pm.

Withdrawal of corticosteroids

Some situations require gradual withdraw of systemic corticosteroids in order to avoid relapse of disease and adrenal failure. These include when the patient has:

- recently repeated steroid courses (particularly if taken for >3 weeks)

- taken a short course within 1 year of stopping long-term therapy

- other possible causes of adrenal suppression

Table 1. Equivalent anti-inflammatory doses of corticosteroids.

Drug	Equivalent anti-inflammatory dose (mg)
Betamethasone	0.75
Cortisone acetate	25
Deflazacort	6
Dexamethasone	0.75
Fludrocortisone	Mineralocorticoid, so no anti-inflammatory activity
Hydrocortisone	20
Methylprednisolone	4
Prednisolone	5
Prednisone	5
Triamcinolone	4

- received prednisolone >40 mg daily (or equivalent)

- taken repeated doses in the evening

- received >3 weeks of corticosteroid treatment

You can reduce the corticosteroid dose rapidly down to the equivalent of prednisolone 7.5 mg daily, but then take withdrawal more slowly.

Example

Remembering to be *C*lear with timing (si*C*kly), reduce from prednisolone 40 mg OD as follows:

- 30 mg OM for 3 days, then...

- ...20 mg OM for 3 days, then...

- ...10 mg OM for 3 days, then...

- ...7.5 mg OM for 5 days, then...

- ...5 mg OM for 5 days, then...

- ...2.5 mg OM for 5 days, then...

- ...stop!

Assess the disease during withdrawal to ensure that relapse does not occur and watch for symptoms of adrenal failure.

You can stop systemic corticosteroids abruptly in those whose disease is unlikely to relapse, and in those who have received treatment for ≤3 weeks and who are not included in the patient groups mentioned previously.

Infections

3

Peter Wilson

Your *choice of antibiotic* should be dictated by spectrum of activity, tissue penetration, potency, cost and local patterns of infection in your hospital. Too much to remember? Ask your microbiologist, who will have written a local antibiotic policy (eg, 'what is first line for hospital-acquired pneumonia?').

If the patient is ill enough to have required admission for the treatment of an infection, the *route of administration* should generally be IV. This ensures that adequate plasma levels are achieved independent of GI absorption. The *dose* should always be checked in the *BNF*.

TOP TIPS for optimising the initial choice of antibiotic

- Take microbiological specimens before starting treatment.

- Base your initial choice of antibiotic on the most likely pathogen(s).

- In the critically ill, use the highest IV dose, but *not* the IM route.

- Be familiar with the *Control of Infection Manual* and the *Hospital Formulary*.

- Microbiology and infection control staff are usually available on 24-hour call. Use them!

Table 2. Treatment options for meningitis.

Infection	Treatment
Covering *S. pneumoniae*, *H. influenzae* and *N. meningitidis*	Ceftriaxone 2 g IV 24-hourly
	For patients with a history of anaphylaxis to penicillins and/or cephalosporins, give chloramphenicol 1 g PO/IV 6- to 8-hourly
For contacts: prophylaxis required	*N. meningitidis*: ciprofloxacin PO one dose or rifampicin PO BD for 2 days
	H. influenzae: ciprofloxacin PO BD for 3 days or rifampicin PO BD for 4 days

If in doubt, *seek advice*! The microbiologists welcome clinical queries – asking a question now can prevent a lot of problems later on.

Antibiotic treatment

Acute meningitis
The antibiotics used to treat meningitis are given in **Table 2**.

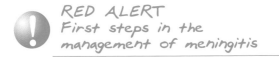

RED ALERT
First steps in the
management of meningitis

- *Do not delay treatment*, particularly if outside a hospital.

- *Do not* wait for a lumbar puncture or CT scan.

- But *do* try to get a blood culture first.

Table 3. Antibiotic options for upper respiratory tract infections.

Infection	Treatment
Acute streptococcal pharyngitis	If admitted: benzylpenicillin IV 6-hourly
	If an oral regimen is to be used: benzylpenicillin IM for one dose then amoxicillin PO 8-hourly for 10 days
	If allergic to penicillin: erythromycin PO for 10 days
Acute otitis media, *S. pneumoniae*, *H. influenzae*	First choice: amoxicillin PO 8-hourly for 5 days
	Or: co-amoxiclav PO 8-hourly for 5 days
	If allergic to penicillin: erythromycin PO for 5 days

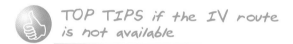

TOP TIPS *if the IV route is not available*

If there is no venous access, give ceftriaxone IM (in more than one site) for the *first dose only*.

• Contact the on-call microbiologist for treatment advice.

• *Do not* administer antibiotics intrathecally.

• Treatment should be modified according to microbiology results.

Remember: this is a notifiable disease. You *must* contact microbiology, who will arrange prophylaxis for all of the patient's home and work contacts.

Upper respiratory tract infections

• These are generally viral and don't usually require antibiotics (see **Table 3**).

• Remember, amoxicillin + glandular fever = rash and unscathed virus!

Table 4. Treatment options for community-acquired pneumonia.

Infection	Treatment
If not severely ill, cover *H. influenzae*, *S. pneumoniae* and atypicals	Amoxicillin PO 8-hourly plus erythromycin PO or amoxicillin IV 8-hourly plus clarithromycin IV 12-hourly
If severely ill, use highest recommended dose IV	First choice: cefuroxime IV 8-hourly plus clarithromycin IV 12-hourly for 7–10 days (may be longer if *Legionella*, staphylococcal or Gram-negative bacilli pneumonia are suspected or confirmed; discuss with microbiology)
Post-influenza: cover against *S. aureus*	As above Cover against *S. aureus* should be adequate with erythromycin, but change to high-dose flucloxacillin if confirmed
Mycoplasma or *Chlamydia* species suspected	Erythromycin or doxycycline
Legionnaire's suspected	Consult a microbiologist urgently!

Lower respiratory tract infections

- Lobar pneumonia in a younger person should be treated more aggressively if there is deterioration on oral agents.

- Empyema is serious. It requires immediate large-bore drainage and possibly surgery. Get specialist advice *at once.*

- Give antibiotics as soon as pneumonia is diagnosed.

- Use IV treatment if the patient has two of:

  – respiratory rate ≥30 breaths/minute

  – diastolic BP ≤60 mm Hg

  – blood urea ≥7 mmol/L

- Clarithromycin causes less GI motility/discomfort than erythromycin.

Community-acquired pneumonia

This is usually susceptible to first-line treatments (see **Table 4**).

Table 5. Treatment options for infective exacerbations of COPD.

Infection	Treatment
Change in sputum colour or volume, or if pyrexial	Cefuroxime IV 8-hourly for the first 48 hours, then amoxicillin PO 8-hourly If allergic to penicillin: doxycycline PO 12- to 24-hourly
More severe exacerbation/poor response to agents above	Consider adding erythromycin PO

Table 6. Treatment options for aspiration pneumonia.

Infection	Treatment
Often mouth flora, ie, anaerobes and microaerophilic streptococci	Co-amoxiclav PO/IV 8-hourly. Clindamycin is too expensive for first-line use If allergic to penicillin: clindamycin 300 mg PO 6-hourly

Table 7. Treatment options for hospital-acquired pneumonia.

Infection	Treatment
Often coliforms, which can be multiresistant	First choice: cefuroxime IV 8-hourly or co-amoxiclav PO/IV 8-hourly
If sensitivity pattern warrants (eg, *Pseudomonas* species) or ventilated on ICU	Ceftazidime IV 8-hourly, piperacillin/tazobactam IV 8-hourly or ciprofloxacin (use 400 mg not 200 mg) IV 12-hourly

Infective exacerbation of COPD

This is usually viral, but it is difficult to distinguish from bacterial (see **Table 5**).

Aspiration pneumonia

Only use antibiotics if there are signs of infection (see **Table 6**).

Hospital-acquired pneumonia

Onset is >72 hours after admission. See **Table 7** for treatment.

TOP TIPS for monitoring patients with hospital-acquired pneumonia

- The need for IV therapy should be reviewed after 48 hours.

- If the patient fails to respond to treatment, take advice from a microbiologist and/or chest physician.

- Remember to consider tuberculosis, HIV infection and underlying diseases such as lung cancer.

Gastroenteritis

- Antibiotics should usually be avoided and can prolong excretion of the pathogen. They *should* be used in patients with typhoid, septicaemia or AIDS (see **Table 8**).

- For other infections, antibiotics should be reserved for the severely ill, immunocompromised or elderly.

- The most important aspect of treatment is oral rehydration with glucose electrolyte solutions (or salty soups and fruit juices) and complex carbohydrates (promote active glucose/sodium co-transport).

- Avoid opioids and loperamide.

TOP TIPS for managing Clostridium difficile (pseudomembranous colitis)

- If the patient is unable to take medication orally, give metronidazole IV 8-hourly (note: IV vancomycin is not effective).

- Persistence of toxin is not a guide to treatment duration.

Table 8. Treatment options for gastroenteritis.

Infection	Treatment
Typhoid	First choice: ciprofloxacin PO/IV 12-hourly or chloramphenicol PO/IV 6-hourly
Salmonella, Shigella	First choice: ciprofloxacin PO/IV 12-hourly
	Alternatives: amoxicillin, tetracycline, chloramphenicol, etc., depending on antibiotic sensitivities. See *BNF* for doses
Campylobacter (treatment often ineffective)	First choice: erythromycin PO
	Alternative: ciprofloxacin PO 12-hourly
Amoebiasis	Metronidazole or tinidazole (single dose at night)
	Diloxanide furoate – on expert advice only
	Avoid steroids
Giardia	Metronidazole, tinidazole or mepacrine hydrochloride (unlicensed product)
Yersinia	Seek expert advice
Cryptosporidiosis	Seek expert advice
Clostridium difficile (pseudomembranous colitis)	This is the most common infective diarrhoea in hospitals
	It is most commonly induced by clindamycin, although most antibiotics can be implicated
	Stop all antibiotics if possible
	If treatment of a concurrent infection is essential, use the antibiotic that is least likely to worsen diarrhoea (eg, ciprofloxacin, vancomycin)
Persisting or severe symptoms	First choice: metronidazole PO 8-hourly (stop before 2 weeks of therapy, as risk of peripheral neuropathy)
	Alternative: vancomycin 125 mg PO 6-hourly (can predispose to the emergence of vancomycin-resistant enterococci)

- Usually, treat established pseudomembranous colitis until diarrhoea stops.

- Surgery might be required. Relapses are common.

Table 9. Treatment options for cellulitis.

Condition	Treatment
First choice	Benzylpenicillin IV 6-hourly + flucloxacillin IV 6-hourly
No IV access	Clindamycin PO 6-hourly
Allergic to penicillin	Clindamycin PO 6-hourly, clarithromycin IV 12-hourly, erythromycin PO or teicoplanin/vancomycin

Cellulitis

- This is a soft-tissue infection.

- Administer IV antibiotics *without delay* for any spreading cellulitis (see **Table 9**).

- Oral treatment is reserved for localised or minor infections.

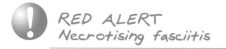

RED ALERT
Necrotising fasciitis

- Blistering, dusky purple or black discolouration suggests necrosis requiring surgical intervention.

- Necrotising fasciitis is a surgical emergency. It is signified by a brown serous discharge, not pus. Seek *immediate* surgical review. *Do not* wait until the morning!

Urinary tract infections

- Upper UTI – give IV antibiotics for 48 hours, then PO for 1 week.

- Lower UTI – give oral treatment for 3 days only. Recurrent infections require longer courses of treatment for 2–6 weeks.

- Complicated infection (eg, anatomical abnormality of the renal tract) – treatment courses should be for 5–7 days (see **Table 10**).

Table 10. Treatment options for UTIs.

Infection	Treatment
Uncomplicated, community acquired	Treat only if symptomatic
	First choice: trimethoprim 200 mg PO 12-hourly
	Alternative: nitrofurantoin 50 mg PO 6-hourly
Hospital acquired	First choice: trimethoprim 200 mg PO 12-hourly
	Alternative: cefuroxime 750 mg IV 8-hourly or nitrofurantoin 50 mg PO 6-hourly
In pregnancy	*Always* treat, even if asymptomatic
	Seek advice from an obstetrician ± microbiologist
	Cefadroxil PO 12-hourly or amoxicillin PO 8-hourly
	Avoid trimethoprim in the first trimester and nitrofurantoin in the last trimester

- Do not treat asymptomatic, elderly or catheterised patients.

- Sexually transmitted diseases can cause similar symptoms, so collect a urinary specimen before treatment whenever practicable.

Bacterial endocarditis

- Always consult the on-call microbiologist. *Do not* try to treat this condition without advice.

- Three separate sets of blood cultures should be taken before starting treatment.

Septicaemia

- Treat *immediately* (see **Table 11**).

- Patients can succumb to Gram-negative bacteraemia if not adequately treated within 12 hours. The urinary, biliary and respiratory tracts are the most likely sources.

Table 11. Treatment options for septicaemia.

Condition	Treatment
Initially	Cefuroxime IV 8-hourly
If patient deteriorates further	Add gentamicin IV
If allergic to cephalosporins	Ciprofloxacin IV 12-hourly + gentamicin IV
If you suspect anaerobic sepsis	Add metronidazole IV 8-hourly

Neutropenic sepsis

- Untreated, these patients deteriorate fast – a single spike of fever is sufficient. Hit Gram-negative pathogens first, then after 24 hours staphylococci and, after a further 24 hours, fungi.

- Check your local hospital protocol.

- The protocol will usually include broad-spectrum antibiotics with activity against *Pseudomonas*.

- If fever is associated with flushing of the Hickman line or redness/discharge around the line exit site, add vancomycin or teicoplanin. Think about taking the line out.

MRSA

MRSA is the most common nosocomial pathogen in an increasing number of hospitals and is readily transmitted on the hands. It might be four times more invasive than methicillin-sensitive *S. aureus*. It is difficult to treat because it is usually resistant to several families of antibiotics. Deep surgical wound infections are particularly troublesome. Prolonged treatment with glycopeptides combined with rifampicin, fusidic acid or gentamicin (depending on susceptibility) is effective in some cases, but surgical debridement is often needed. Metal or plastic work must be removed for cure.

Antibiotic prophylaxis

General principles

- In most surgical specialties, antibiotic prophylaxis has been shown to be effective in reducing post-operative wound infections.

- It is not needed in minor clean procedures (eg, simple hernia repair, removal of lipoma).

- Parenteral antibiotics should be given with induction of anaesthesia before skin incision. Tissue levels will then be sufficient to kill the bacteria (see **Table 12**).

- Antibiotics given >4 hours after surgery are *not* an effective prevention.

- A single large dose of antibiotic is sufficient, except in vascular, head and neck surgery.

- If infection still results, use a different antibiotic to treat the infection from the one used for prophylaxis.

TOP TIPS for the administration of prophylactic antibiotics

- Ensure that administration is always documented (this is a medico-legal requirement).

- Adjust the dose if the patient is obese.

- Do not give antibiotics with premedication because the timing is variable.

- Check whether the patient has had any recent infections with resistant organisms.

- Eradicate MRSA carriage using topical therapy (chlorhexidine, mupirocin nasal ointment) before surgery or, if an emergency, during the peri-operative period.

Table 12. Prophylactic antibiotic choices prior to surgery. *Continued opposite.*

GI procedures	
Appendectomy	Cefuroxime and metronidazole IV
	If the appendix is acutely inflamed or if pus is found, continue with cefuroxime IV 8-hourly + metronidazole IV 8-hourly for 5 days
Colorectal surgery	Cefuroxime + metronidazole IV
Biliary tract surgery	
Normal bile duct, no stents	No prophylaxis needed
Cholecystectomy, biliary tree involvement, common duct stones	First choice: cefuroxime Alternative: co-amoxiclav Allergic to penicillin: ciprofloxacin
Previous biliary surgery	Add gentamicin IV to the above
Anaerobes suspected, eg, carcinoma	Add metronidazole IV to cefuroxime No need to add metronidazole to co-amoxiclav
Upper GI surgery	Cefuroxime IV
	For anhydric patients/those with gastro-oesophageal cancer, add metronidazole IV
Vascular procedures	
First choice	Cefuroxime IV
Second choice	Co-amoxiclav 1.2 g IV at induction
Allergic to penicillin	Clarithromycin IV
MRSA	Teicoplanin or vancomycin used with gentamicin
Gynaecological procedures	
Hysterectomy, emergency Caesarean section	First choice: co-amoxiclav IV
	Allergic to penicillin: clindamycin IV
Termination of pregnancy	Uncomplicated: no prophylactic antibiotic
	History of pelvic inflammatory disease: doxycycline 100 mg BD for 10 days post-operatively
Orthopaedic procedures	
Compound fracture	Benzylpenicillin IV at induction, then IV/IM 6-hourly thereafter
	At 24–48 hours, switch to penicillin V PO 6-hourly, as indicated by clinical situation

Table 12. *Continued.*

Joint replacement and spinal surgery	First choice: cefuroxime IV at induction, then (if prosthesis inserted) IV 8-hourly for two doses; or flucloxacillin IV at induction, then (if prosthesis inserted) PO 6-hourly for two doses
	Allergic to penicillin: clarithromycin IV at induction, then (if prosthesis inserted) erythromycin PO 6-hourly for two doses
	For infected joint replacement, start specific treatment rather than giving antibiotic prophylaxis
	For repeat procedures due to infection, gentamicin cement should be incorporated during the procedure
	Metronidazole is *not* indicated for routine orthopaedic prophylaxis
Urological procedures	
Mid-stream urine culture must be checked before and during surgery	
Transrectal prostatic biopsy	First choice: gentamicin IV + metronidazole suppository before procedure
	Second choice: ciprofloxacin 500 mg PO 1–2 hours before procedure

4

Therapeutic Drug Monitoring

Nicola Mayne

It might sound dull, but it is crucial that you understand TDM: *failure = worse treatments and severe toxicity!*

Drugs that are suitable for TDM have a recognised desired serum concentration range. Within this range, the drug will produce its optimal effect with minimal toxicity. TDM is therefore necessary for two reasons:

1. To determine whether the drug is at therapeutic plasma concentrations – for most drugs, the easiest way to determine efficacy is by achieving a clinical endpoint. However, for certain drugs, TDM is the only way to ensure that your drug is working (are you really preventing the next fit?).

2. To determine if the drug is at toxic levels – some drugs have a 'narrow therapeutic range', where the difference between efficacious and toxic concentrations is small. TDM aids drug dosing, keeping plasma levels within the desired efficacious range and out of the toxic range.

For every drug that you prescribe, think sick*L*y – *L*evels! The drugs that you are most likely to encounter that require TDM are gentamicin, phenytoin, digoxin and theophylline/aminophylline. When you're thinking about measuring a level, you need to know the following...

Why you are measuring a drug level?

- Are you interested in achieving a therapeutic target, avoiding the toxic range or both?

- Do you suspect a drug interaction? The drugs mentioned are prone to multiple drug interactions. Revise your enzyme inducers and inhibitors!

- Have you noted a decline in renal or hepatic function? The drugs mentioned are either renally excreted (gentamicin) or hepatically metabolised (phenytoin, digoxin, theophylline), so be extra vigilant with levels if renal or hepatic function declines.

When to measure the drug level

A level taken at random is no help to anyone. It takes about 4–5 half-lives for a regularly administered drug to accumulate in the blood, at which point the drug is said to be in steady state. Once the drug has reached steady state, you either take a…

- …*trough level*, ie, sample immediately before the dose is due, when the drug concentration is at its lowest, or a…

- …*peak level* – timing depends on the half-life of a drug – the longer the half-life, the longer you have to wait before the drug concentration is at its highest

What the results mean

Remember to label the sample with the *time of sampling* and the *time of dosing*. Without this information, the lab staff cannot help you to interpret the result.

How to act on what you find

This is not always simple. When in doubt, get help!

But before considering anything complex, ask yourself some simple questions:

- Is there a compliance issue that you can deal with?

- Is there a possible drug interaction?

If the latter, see if you can find an alternative to the offending drug. If there is no alternative, but the offending drug is for a short course (eg, antibiotics), then continue with both drugs, monitor for signs of drug failure or toxicity and recheck levels when the offending drug is stopped.

If there is no alternative, but the offending drug is needed for a more chronic duration, seek expert advice.

Common examples

Gentamicin

Be aware of the two methods of gentamicin dosing – the 'conventional' method and the 'once-daily' method (see **Table 13**).

Pay particular attention to older patients whose kidneys have seen better days. These patients are most likely to require a dose adjustment. On the flip side, the higher the peak the faster the kill, so *ad hoc* dose reductions are not the answer.

Table 13. Gentamicin TDM.

Conventional dosing	
Dose	1–1.5 mg/kg IV with frequency depending on estimated creatinine clearance. If creatinine clearance: • >70 mL/minute, 8-hourly • 30–70 mL/minute, 12-hourly • 10–30 mL/minute, 24-hourly • 5–10 mL/minute, 48-hourly
Why?	To avoid toxicity
When?	Take a trough level before the third dose or on day 2
Meaning?	The trough level should be <2 mg/mL
Action?	If the trough level is >2 mg/mL, withhold doses until the level falls to <2 mg/mL Adjust the dosage interval rather than the actual dose
Once-daily dosing	
Dose	5 or 7 mg/kg IV If the patient is obese, do not use their actual weight, but calculate their corrected body weight (see p. 196)
Why?	To avoid toxicity
When?	Take levels any time between 6 and 14 hours post-dose
Meaning?	Refer to the Hartford nomogram (see **Figure 1**)
Action?	If the levels are high, increase the interval between doses as per the Hartford nomogram
Note	Once-daily dosing is not appropriate in patients who have creatinine clearance <20 mL/minute, endocarditis, severe liver disease, cystic fibrosis or major burns, or for prophylaxis or in infants <6 months

Figure 1. The Hartford nomogram.

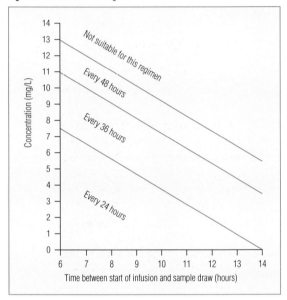

Important calculations:
For obese patients, use
corrected body weight

- Ideal body weight (IBW):

    IBW (male) = 50 kg in weight +
    (2.3 × every inch over 5 ft in height)

    IBW (female) = 45 kg in weight +
    (2.3 × every inch over 5 ft in height)

- Excess body weight (EBW):

    EBW (kg) = actual body weight – IBW

    $\% \text{ Obesity} = \dfrac{\text{actual body weight} - \text{IBW}}{\text{IBW}} \times 100$

- Corrected body weight (CBW):

$$CBW \ (kg) = IBW + (0.4 \times EBW)$$

Use if patient is >15% obese.

Digoxin
See **Table 14**.

Key drugs that can increase digoxin levels

- Amiodarone
- Bendroflumethiazide
- Ciclosporin
- Diltiazem
- Furosemide
- Itraconazole
- Macrolides
- Propafenone
- Quinidine
- Spironolactone
- Telmisartan
- Verapamil

Key drugs that can reduce digoxin levels

- Antacids
- Colestyramine
- St John's wort

Phenytoin
See **Table 15** (p. 199).

Key drugs that can increase phenytoin levels

- Amiodarone
- Chloramphenicol
- Cimetidine
- Clarithromycin
- Fluconazole
- Fluvoxamine
- Isoniazid
- Metronidazole
- Trimethoprim
- Voriconazole

Key drugs that can reduce phenytoin levels

- Alcohol
- Antacids
- Carbamazepine
- Rifampicin
- St John's wort
- Theophylline

Table 14. Digoxin TDM. *Continued opposite.*

Loading dose	Urgent: 0.75–1 mg IV over 2 hours or 1–1.5 mg PO over 24 hours in divided doses Less urgent: 250–500 μg PO daily for 3 days
Maintenance dose	125–250 μg PO OD Less in the elderly or the renally impaired
Why?	To avoid toxicity To investigate treatment failure
When?	Take levels 1 week after starting treatment Sample pre-dose or 6–9 hours post-dose Not necessary in all patients starting therapy – advisable in the elderly and the renally impaired
Meaning?	Recommended therapeutic range: • 0.5–0.8 μg/L target in heart failure • 1.5–2 μg/L target in arrhythmia >3 μg/L is usually associated with signs of toxicity Toxicity is possible at levels as low as 1.5 μg/L
Action?	Patient toxic and levels raised: • if life-threatening (ie, level >4 μg/L), omit drug and treat with Digibind® • determine cause before restarting • if restarting, consider a lower dose. In general, to achieve a serum concentration of half the value, reduce the maintenance dose by half Patient toxic but levels within therapeutic range: • exclude other causes of toxic symptoms • check K⁺ • reduce dose, consider additional therapy for cardiac failure or arrhythmia Patient clinically undertreated and levels low: • increase dose, usually by 50–75 μg, and recheck levels

Table 14. *Continued.*

	Patient clinically undertreated, but levels within therapeutic range: • consider additional therapy
Important!	Hypokalaemia and hypothyroidism are commonly associated with digoxin toxicity so, in suspected toxicity, check K⁺ and thyroid function!

Table 15. Phenytoin TDM. *Continued overleaf.*

Loading dose	15 mg/kg IV: maximum rate of 50 mg/minute
Maintenance dose	100 mg IV 6- to 8-hourly
	150–300 mg PO OD, gradually increasing to 200–500 mg PO OD
	Doses can be split if not tolerated
Why?	To ensure you are achieving the therapeutic target
	To avoid toxicity
	Phenytoin has a narrow therapeutic index
	A fit-free patient, with no signs of toxicity, requires no levels
When?	Take levels 2–4 weeks after starting the drug or changing the dose
	For IV therapy: 4–6 hours post-dose
	For PO therapy: trough level pre-dose
	In an emergency, take levels at any time
Meaning?	Recommended therapeutic range: 40–80 μmol/L or 10–20 mg/L
	The drug is largely albumin bound, so you might need to adjust for a low albumin:
	adjusted phenytoin level = reported level $\div$ ([0.02 × serum albumin {g/L}] + 0.1)

Table 15. *Continued.*

Action?	Patient showing toxic signs and level raised or within range:
	• seek expert advice on dose reduction
	Patient fitting and levels low:
	• seek expert advice on repeating a loading dose
	• increase maintenance dose as follows:
	– <28 µmol/L level, increase daily dose by 100 mg OD
	– 28–48 µmol/L level, increase daily dose by 50 mg OD
	– 48–64 µmol/L level, increase daily dose by 25 mg OD
	Patient fitting and levels in therapeutic range:
	• seek expert advice – the patient might well need additional/alternative therapy
	Before you make a dose change, seek expert advice!

Table 16. Theophylline/aminophylline TDM. *Continued opposite.*

Loading dose	Aminophylline 5 mg/kg IV over 20 minutes
Maintenance dose	Aminophylline 500 µg/kg/hour IV titrated to plasma levels
	Oral therapy depends on the brand
	In obese patients, use ideal body weight to calculate the dose – aminophylline distributes poorly in adipose tissue
Why?	To ensure you are achieving the therapeutic target
	To avoid toxicity
	For IV therapy: TDM is essential, as the drug has a narrow therapeutic range
	For PO therapy: TDM is not generally required unless the patient is clinically undertreated or showing signs of toxicity
When?	For IV therapy: take levels at 1 and 6 hours, repeating daily
	For PO therapy: take trough levels after 2–3 days of treatment

Table 16. *Continued.*

Meaning?	Recommended therapeutic range: 55–110 µmol/L or 10–20 mg/L
Action?	In most patients theophylline has linear kinetics, so doubling the dose will double the serum concentration. But look out for the odd patient who breaks the rule!
	Acute patient, with low/high level: • adjust dose by desired fraction
	Acute patient in range: • repeat levels daily
	Chronic patient, with low/high level: • having excluded a reversible cause, adjust the dose
	Chronic patient in range: • suspected toxicity: consider a second drug or pathology causing toxic signs. You might need to stop theophylline regardless
	Symptomatic patient: • consider alternative therapy
Important!	Children metabolise theophylline quicker than adults so are likely to require higher doses.
	Beware of those in whom the theophylline half-life is increased, ie, those in whom a normal dose might cause toxicity: cardiac failure, liver failure, the elderly, those taking enzyme inhibitors (eg, cimetidine, ciprofloxacin)
	Beware of those in whom the theophylline half-life is decreased, ie, those in whom a normal dose might be ineffective: smokers, chronic alcoholics, those taking enzyme inducers (eg, rifampicin, phenytoin). The effect of smoking can be maintained up to 6 months after cessation

Theophylline/aminophylline

See **Table 16**. Serum levels predict the type of adverse effects well, but are less good at predicting severity (see **Table 17**).

Vancomycin

See **Table 18**.

Table 17. Levels associated with adverse effects of aminophylline and theophylline.

Level (mg/L)	Adverse reaction	Frequency (%)
<5	Usually absent	–
5–20	Nausea and vomiting	5–10
20–35	As above + diarrhoea, irritability, arrhythmias	25
>35	As above + seizures	80

Table 18. Vancomycin TDM.

Dose	Usually start at 1 g IV BD
	For the elderly or those with low body weight: 500 mg IV BD
Why?	Vancomycin is renally toxic and ototoxic at raised levels
When?	Take a trough level in the morning before the third or fourth doses, ie, day 2 of treatment. Repeat levels either: • daily if renal function is poor • twice weekly if renal function is stable
Meaning?	Trough level: 5–10 mg/L Peak level: this is not required

Action?	Raised trough level:
	• 11–15 mg/L, reduce dose by 25% (eg, to 750 mg IV BD)
	• 16–20 mg/L, omit the next dose then reduce by 50% (eg, 500 mg IV BD)
	• >20 mg/L, omit drug and repeat level daily
	  – when level <10 mg/L, give 1 g IV
	  – repeat for each dose

Table 19. Other commonly prescribed drugs that require TDM.

Drug	Half-life (hours)	Target range	When to sample and sampling notes
Carbamazepine	Chronic therapy, 5–27	17–50 µmol/L	Trough level after 2–4 weeks
		4–12 mg/L	Aim for higher end of range if monotherapy
			Half-life decreases with chronic therapy
Ciclosporin	9	200–400 µg/L	As per local policy
Lithium	18	0.4–1.3 mmol/L	12 hours post-dose
			Desired level varies with indication
Phenobarbitone	120	65–172 µmol/L	Any time after 3–4 weeks, due to long half-life
		15–40 mg/L	Poor correlation between level and response
Sodium valproate	8–15	350–700 µmol/L	Take trough level after 2–4 days
		50–100 mg/L	Less reliable correlation between level and efficacy

Other drugs

Table 19 gives a summary of some other drugs that you might be asked to check levels for.

5 Drug Hyper-sensitivities and Contraindications

Roman Landowski

Primum non nocere ('first, do no harm') is a fine principle. But any medicine worth using has a risk of side effects, so it is important to assess the risk–benefit ratio.

Being written by lawyers, the manufacturers' data sheets tend to be overly liberal with their contraindications. So how do you make your assessment? Use your pharmacy medicines information centre to understand local and national guidelines and *BNF* guidance – then you won't have to blindly follow the rules, but will be able to use them to guide your particular clinical options.

Enshrined rules and received wisdom tend to fit into one of three categories:

The Good: sensible advice that you should try to follow.

The Bad: overly cautious advice that you can (usually) flout with impunity.

The Ugly: tricky advice that might appear overly cautious, but that you should still follow as it is usually the safer alternative.

The Good

"Don't give him NSAIDs – he's got renal impairment."

Patients with renal impairment rely on renal prostaglandins to maintain their blood flow – and these are blocked by NSAIDs. Therefore, NSAIDs will worsen renal perfusion in these patients and precipitate a sudden deterioration in renal function. Liver failure and heart failure patients might be similarly dependent. COX-2 inhibitors (eg, celecoxib, etoricoxib) are just as bad and you should avoid them all. Use paracetamol, tramadol or opioids as alternative analgesics.

"Don't use NSAIDs in liver failure."

Bleeding is a common problem in decompensated liver disease and NSAIDs can exacerbate this (anti-platelet effects) or cause bleeding (GI ulcers). In this regard the COX-2 inhibitors are better, but they can still cause GI bleeding. So avoid the lot and stick to paracetamol/tramadol for pain and prednisolone for inflammation.

"Avoid morphine and central nervous system depressants in liver failure."

The worry here is tipping your patient into hepatic encephalopathy. Remember, though, that the central nervous system-depressant effects of opioids (and of any drug) are dose dependent. So morphine can be used to treat severe pain in cirrhosis as long as you start at low doses (eg, 5 mg PO) and increase in small increments, and only as long as the patient is conscious enough to appreciate it!

With anti-histamines, obviously try the non-sedating loratadine or cetirizine first. If you need to use a stronger anti-pruritic such as chlorpheniramine or hydroxyzine then start with a half dose and increase as tolerated.

The Bad

"Beta-blockers kill asthmatics."

Well yes, it can happen, but the risk depends on the degree of beta-2 blockade (bronchial effect) that you inflict. Cardioselective beta-blockers (eg, atenolol, bisoprolol) mainly block beta-1 (cardiac) receptors (although you might see asthma exacerbation at high doses). Non-selective beta-blockers (eg, propranolol, carvedilol) are more likely to cause bronchoconstriction, especially at high doses. So, you can use beta-blockers safely in non-brittle asthmatics if you stick to the cardioselective ones – start at low doses and watch out for signs of asthma exacerbation whenever you increase the dose.

"Don't use cephalosporins in patients allergic to penicillin!"

OK, so cephalosporins and penicillin are both beta-lactams and there is a recognised cross-allergy, which books will tell you is 10%. Half of the problem is that people describe non-immunological reactions such as headache, confusion and diarrhoea as evidence of allergy. They might well be hypersensitivity reactions, but they are not allergic.

If the patient is sure that he/she has had a real immunological reaction such as oedema or rash then try to use a non-cephalosporin alternative (eg, gentamicin for UTIs or clarithromycin for chest infections). Otherwise, check that the emergency tray is in date and crack on with the cefuroxime!

"Aspirin with warfarin is dangerous."

Correction: warfarin is dangerous however you prescribe it – it features in half of all hospital adverse incident reports. Aspirin is often co-prescribed with warfarin for the treatment of a venous or arterial thrombosis. The problem arises when patients self-medicate with PRN aspirin, as the high doses used for pain relief (eg, 600 mg QDS) are much more likely to cause bleeds than low anti-platelet doses (eg, 75 mg OD). Regular anti-platelet aspirin is not without risk, but it is at least predictable, monitorable and reducible (with concomitant omeprazole).

The Ugly

"Better stop the metformin as he is now in renal failure."

Tricky – does renal failure really increase your risk of lactic acidosis with metformin? A 2006 Cochrane review concluded that the evidence was thin. The trouble is that this very rare side effect has a high mortality (approximately 50%), and the benefit of the drug probably doesn't justify the worry involved in prescribing it. Change to a glitazone or just ask the patient to inject insulin.

"Young girls can't take metoclopramide."

There is an element of truth in this. Teenage girls seem to be particularly prone to extra-pyramidal reactions caused by dopamine antagonists such as metoclopramide. These Parkinsonian reactions are not dangerous, but they are distressing for the patient. Of course, most girls won't have this reaction and, as it is dose-related, you can try using a half dose first. Still, the whole point of giving metoclopramide is to stop nausea, which is less likely to occur if you are using homeopathic doses, so it's easier to just use cyclizine or domperidone first and then granisetron if things don't improve.

"Don't give aspirin to asthmatics."

Aspirin is said to set off asthma in about 5% of asthmatics and, although this effect is dose-related, it often occurs at low doses (an average of 69 mg in one study). If the patient has had previous aspirin or NSAIDs without bronchoconstriction then you can be sure that they won't react now. If you're starting low-dose aspirin in a patient who is unsure whether he/she has had aspirin or NSAIDs before, start at a quarter of a 75-mg tablet for the first dose, then half a tablet and then a full tablet on day 3. If there are any problems then convert to clopidogrel.

Likewise, if you need immediate anti-platelet effects then give a loading dose (300 mg) of clopidogrel and then titrate up the aspirin. NSAIDs show the same problem as aspirin, but COX-2 inhibitors are safe, so use celecoxib if your asthmatic patient needs an anti-inflammatory.

The ridiculous!

"He can't have penicillamine because he's allergic to penicillin."

Yes, penicillamine is a breakdown product of penicillin and yes, the spellings are quite similar, but no, penicillamine does not have a beta-lactam ring and cross-hypersensitivity is very much the exception rather than the rule.

Interactions that Matter

Roman Landowski

The man lay on our renal ward, too weak to rise, limbs aching, new bedsores burning and his transplant failing. Two lines on his drug chart explained why:

1. Ciclosporin 100 mg BD (but he had been on that uneventfully for years).

2. He recently started simvastatin 20 mg ON.

And there it was – iatrogenic rhabdomyolysis from a simple drug interaction.

How do drugs interact?

Pharmacokinetic interactions

- Enzyme inhibition – eg, as above, ciclosporin inhibits the simvastatin-metabolising cytochrome P450 3A4, causing simvastatin levels to double and the risk of (level-dependent) rhabdomyolysis to rise.

- Enzyme induction – eg, rifampicin can induce P450 C9, which metabolises warfarin. Result? The warfarin levels are halved and the INR is reduced to ineffective levels unless the warfarin dose is doubled. Unlike enzyme inhibition, which occurs soon after the interacting drug is added, the effects of enzyme induction can take a couple of weeks to reach their peak.

- Reduced absorption – eg, calcium taken with ciprofloxacin binds to form an insoluble chelate, lowering ciprofloxacin blood levels. Avoid by leaving a 2-hour time gap between the drugs.

- Competition for renal excretion, raising the levels of each drug – eg, probenecid raises amoxicillin levels by a factor of 2- to 4-fold, so when treating endocarditis use amoxicillin 500 mg PO QDS + probenecid 500 mg PO QDS.

- Drug displacement from protein binding sites (usually on albumin) – this rarely has clinical consequences. Valproate can displace phenytoin from albumin binding sites, but the rise in free phenytoin is temporary as it is free phenytoin that is cleared. Since a greater amount is available for clearance, the free phenytoin will return to normal (although it will be a larger proportion of the total phenytoin, which will itself have fallen).

Pharmacodynamic interactions

In these interactions, two drugs either have opposing effects on the same receptor (eg, propranolol and salbutamol on bronchial beta-2 receptors) or they share common side effects (eg, ciclosporin and simvastatin independently cause an increased risk of myopathy – this is a second reason for the interaction in the opening paragraph).

An approach to interactions

Appendix 1 in the *BNF* gives a good list of potential drug interactions. However, they aren't all clinically relevant – some are theoretical and rarely seen (eg, amiodarone–amitriptyline), while others are simply very rare (eg, phenytoin–digoxin).

The more serious interactions usually involve those drugs where levels need to be increased only *slightly* above their therapeutic range for toxicity to occur. These drugs are commonly

Table 20. Drugs that require monitoring as elevated levels can cause toxicity.

Drugs that require monitoring			
Carbamazepine	Digoxin	Phenytoin	Theophylline
Ciclosporin	Lithium	Statins	Warfarin

Table 21. Drugs that are commonly involved in increasing or decreasing plasma levels.

Drugs likely to cause interactions	
Enzyme inhibitors likely to increase levels	**Enzyme inducers likely to reduce levels**
Ciprofloxacin	Carbamazepine
Diltiazem	Phenobarbitone
Erythromycin	Rifampicin
Fluconazole	St John's wort
Ritonavir	

monitored (see **Chapter 6** of this section). *Think*, is your drug one of these? Examples are given in **Table 20**.

Next, you should check whether any drug that is recognised to cause interactions has been prescribed. Examples of these are given in **Table 21**.

It's back to si*C*kly – if the drug that you intend to prescribe falls into any of these categories then you should actively *C*heck for interactions.

 TOP TIPS for reference sources to check for drug interactions

- Appendix 1 of the *BNF*.

- *Stockley's Drug Interactions*.

- Your ward pharmacist or pharmacy medicines information centre.

In summary, remember your *M*edicines *I*nformation *C*entre – if you are prescribing a drug that requires *M*onitoring or is known to cause frequent *I*nteractions then *C*heck to see whether any problems are likely to be caused by your new drug interacting with what is already on the patient's drug chart!

Specific examples

Warfarin has so many drug interactions that it deserves a chapter to itself, so we gave it one (see **Section 5**, **Chapter 1**). For other drugs, we have detailed the more common interactions that are both predictable and serious. The drug affected is named first in **bold** with the interacting drug next in blue, and this is followed by a summary of the effects, mechanism and recommendations for use in practice.

Alendronate – Calcium

Alendronate and other bisphosphonates such as **clodronate** and **risedronate** work by chelating calcium in bone, where they inhibit bone turnover. They will also chelate ingested calcium taken at the same time, and so become unavailable for absorption. To avoid this, allow a 30-minute gap between any calcium supplements or milk and the oral bisphosphonate.

Azathioprine – Allopurinol

Azathioprine levels increase by a factor of 3–4 after allopurinol is started. This can lead to azathioprine-induced neutropenia and thrombocytopenia (dose related). Allopurinol inhibits xanthine oxidase, which is the enzyme responsible for clearing azathioprine. If azathioprine is being started in a patient already on allopurinol, prescribe one quarter to one third of the usual dose. Xanthine oxidase also clears **mercaptopurine**, so a similar dose reduction is required when allopurinol is added.

Carbamazepine – Erythromycin

Erythromycin and, to a lesser extent, clarithromycin inhibit carbamazepine metabolism, increasing the levels of carbamazepine by 2- to 4-fold. Symptoms of toxicity (ataxia, nausea, confusion, double vision and AV block) develop over 1–3 days. If alternative antibiotics can't be used then you should monitor carbamazepine levels and adjust the dose accordingly. Once erythromycin is stopped, the carbamazepine levels will fall over about a week. Azithromycin does not interact with carbamazepine.

Ciclosporin – Phenytoin

Ciclosporin levels halve over 2 weeks after phenytoin has been added, necessitating an approximate doubling of the ciclosporin dosage. When starting phenytoin in a patient already on ciclosporin, check the ciclosporin levels twice a week and increase the dosage gradually, as necessary. Continue for at least 2 weeks or until dose requirements even out. The same can occur after phenobarbitone or carbamazepine are started.

Ciprofloxacin/Doxycycline – Calcium

Ciprofloxacin (and other quinolones, such as **ofloxacin** and **norfloxacin**) levels drop by 30–50% when calcium is taken at the same time, because calcium chelates ciprofloxacin in the gut. So separate administration by at least 2 hours (and preferably 4 hours).

Tetracyclines such as **doxycycline** or **oxytetracycline** interact likewise and the same rules of separation apply. Iron and antacids containing magnesium or aluminium will also chelate tetracyclines or quinolones if taken at the same time, so should likewise be separated. Milk can also chelate these antibiotics if given in volumes ≥300 mL. The quantities in tea or coffee are unlikely to cause clinical problems.

Digoxin – Amiodarone

Digoxin levels are doubled in some patients when amiodarone is added, due to reduced renal clearance. The effects are nausea, bradycardia, arrhythmias and visual disturbances. These can occur over 7–28 days. Take a level at the beginning of treatment and again after 2 and 4 weeks, and adjust digoxin doses as necessary.

In practice, you would normally halve the digoxin dose immediately upon commencement of amiodarone. If you do this then it is important to check the digoxin level after a month to ensure that the reduction was warranted.

Digoxin – Furosemide

Digoxin toxicity is more likely when patients are hypokalaemic, so beware of digoxin toxicity (in the face of normal levels) when using potassium-losing diuretics such as furosemide and bendroflumethiazide. This problem is less likely if the patient is also taking an ACE inhibitor, an ARB or spironolactone because these all raise potassium. Otherwise, it is better to prescribe co-amilofruse (amiloride with furosemide) than furosemide.

Digoxin – Verapamil

Digoxin levels can be increased in a dose-dependent manner by concurrent verapamil. This can cause digoxin toxicity unless digoxin doses are reduced by 33–50%. Verapamil 160 mg OD increases digoxin levels by 40%, while verapamil 240 mg OD increases levels by 70%. The effect is due to reduced clearance and takes place over 2–14 days. Since verapamil and digoxin share similar slowing effects on the sinoatrial and AV nodes there is an increased risk of bradycardia and AV block, even if digoxin levels remain unchanged. Diltiazem is less likely to increase digoxin levels, so would be a safer alternative to verapamil.

Lithium – Diclofenac

Lithium levels can be raised by 15–60% when NSAIDs such as diclofenac, ibuprofen or indomethacin are added. This is dangerous because lithium toxicity (with its effects of restlessness, nausea and neurotoxicity) occurs just above therapeutic levels (therapeutic: 0.4–1.2 μmol/L; toxic: >1.5 μmol/L). Toxicity, which develops over 1–7 days, is possibly due to NSAID-induced sodium retention (lithium tends to follow sodium in the kidney). Lithium should be monitored at the beginning and after 1 week of concomitant NSAIDs – or sooner if toxicity is suspected.

Methadone – Rifampicin

Enzyme induction means that **methadone** levels can be halved by the concurrent use of rifampicin. To prevent opioid withdrawal, methadone doses should be built up over 2–5 weeks to about 2–3 times the initial dose. Better control can be achieved by splitting the daily dose into two parts to allow for more rapid clearance.

Phenytoin – Nasogastric feeds

Oral **phenytoin** is chelated by nasogastric feeds (but not by normal food), resulting in a potentially large but inconsistent reduction in phenytoin absorption and a fall in the phenytoin level. Stopping the feed for 1 hour before and for 2 hours after phenytoin might help. If not, change to IV phenytoin by giving the preferred daily dose of phenytoin split into 2–4 evenly spread doses (eg, 300 mg NG OD to 100 mg IV TDS).

Prednisolone – Rifampicin/Carbamazepine

Levels of **prednisolone** and other glucocorticoids such as **hydrocortisone** and **dexamethasone** can be reduced 2- to 3-fold by concurrent rifampicin over 2–14 days (due to enzyme induction). This necessitates a 2- to 3-fold increase in steroid dose over about 2 weeks, and a similar tailing off over 2 weeks once the rifampicin is stopped. Carbamazepine affects steroids in the same way.

Simvastatin – Ciclosporin

Simvastatin levels can be doubled by the concomitant use of ciclosporin; this can cause simvastatin-mediated myopathy or rhabdomyolysis. Simvastatin can still be used as long as the dose is restricted to 10 mg/day. Other statins interact similarly, although less so for **pravastatin** and least of all for **fluvastatin**, which is the safest.

Simvastatin – Erythromycin

Simvastatin levels can be increased 3- to 6-fold by macrolides such as clarithromycin, azithromycin or erythromycin. These inhibit 3A4 enzymes, which metabolise simvastatin. Symptoms of myopathy appear in 4–20 days, and it is most simple to stop the statin for the duration of the antibiotic course. If the course is long, either search for an alternative antibiotic or switch to **pravastatin** or **rosuvastatin**, which are less likely to interact.

Simvastatin – Fluconazole

Simvastatin and **atorvastatin** levels can be increased by the triazole anti-fungals fluconazole and itraconazole (enzyme inhibition), leading to a risk of myopathy. For short courses of anti-fungals, stop simvastatin or atorvastatin for the duration. For long courses (over a month), switch to **pravastatin** or **rosuvastatin** (reportedly safe).

Tacrolimus – Erythromycin

Erythromycin, clarithromycin and azithromycin raise **tacrolimus** levels by 4- to 6-fold over 3 days, resulting in tacrolimus toxicity (including renal damage). Levels return to normal just as quickly after erythromycin is stopped, but unless you want to be taking daily tacrolimus levels it is better to swap to another antibiotic (eg, doxycycline). **Ciclosporin** is similarly affected when given with these macrolides.

Theophylline – Ciprofloxacin

Theophylline or **aminophylline** levels can be rapidly increased 2- to 3-fold by concurrent ciprofloxacin (enzyme inhibition). Symptoms of theophylline toxicity (see erythromycin) might well ensue unless theophylline/ aminophylline doses are halved at the onset of ciprofloxacin.

Norfloxacin has less of an effect, while ofloxacin and levofloxacin do not interact.

Theophylline – Erythromycin

Erythromycin will inhibit the 3A4 enzymes that metabolise **theophylline**, leading to a 25–40% increase in theophylline levels after 3–5 days. Once the antibiotics are stopped, it takes about 2 days for theophylline to fall back to its previous level. Check levels at the beginning of therapy, and if they are near the top of the range (>80 µmol/L or 15 mg/L) then shave 25% off the theophylline dose for the duration of the antibiotic course. Otherwise, continue with the normal dose unless symptoms of toxicity (eg, tachycardia, agitation, nausea) occur, in which case withhold theophylline and take levels. The same goes for **aminophylline**.

Azithromycin and clarithromycin are weaker enzyme inhibitors and do not interact to a clinically significant extent with theophylline or aminophylline.

7 Intravenous Therapy

Rob Shulman

Some simple rules!

Rule 1. Check that the patient really needs the IV drug, and can't have it some other (cheaper and less risky) way.

Rule 2. Don't administer an IV drug until you know how. Check your hospital's IV guide or try the appendix of the *BNF*.

Rule 3. Get a check from someone else before you administer the drug. It's been known for tired doctors to read an ampoule as saying 'ampicillin' when it *actually* says 'strong potassium chloride'. *Never trust yourself.* Check the drug, concentration, quantity, expiry date and that you're giving the right drug at the right dose.

Rule 4. Consider whether the IV route should be peripheral or central. See the tips below to take the trauma out of the parenteral route!

Indications for central venous administration

Any of the following can be an indication for the central IV route:

• You are administering hypertonic, concentrated (eg, potassium chloride IV) or irritant fluids (eg, cytotoxics, parenteral nutrition, inotropes).

- You need to rapidly administer large volumes (eg, the patient is in shock).

- You need long-term venous access (eg, cytotoxics).

- You are administering drugs that have a pharmacological action on veins, such as vasoconstriction (eg, dopamine, noradrenaline).

- You need to give incompatible drugs at the same time (central lines can have multiple lumens).

Drugs that *must* be administered centrally include adrenaline, noradrenaline, dopamine and amiodarone infusions.

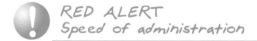

RED ALERT
Speed of administration

Guidelines are there for a reason! Too fast, and…

- furosemide – ototoxicity (deafness) at >4 mg/minute

- fusidic acid – haemolysis and hepatotoxicity

- vancomycin – 'red man' syndrome (flushing, macular rash, fever, rigors), especially if given over <1 hour

- sulphonamides – crystals in the urine

- ranitidine – arrhythmias, arrest

- theophylline – arrhythmias, nausea, vomiting, tachycardia

- potassium chloride – arrhythmias, arrest (generally avoid >20 mM/hour)

- lignocaine – arrhythmias, arrest

- phenytoin – arrhythmias, respiratory/cardiac arrest if administered at >50 mg/minute

- methylprednisolone sodium succinate – cardiovascular collapse at >50 mg/minute

Problems!

Pain on injection

Pain can be caused by factors including pH, tonicity and chemical irritancy.

- Check that you have the right drug. Potassium chloride hurts like hell before it kills you!

- Ensure that the drug is going into the vein and not an artery or tissues!

- Check whether it's a common problem with that particular drug. Pain is seen more with erythromycin, 8.4% $NaHCO_3$, glucose at concentrations >10%, phenytoin and vancomycin.

If the patient is still experiencing pain, try reducing the rate or increasing the dilution.

Phlebitis

This is a red, corded (hard), inflamed vein, with a low flow of drug solution through the vein. Do not plough on – resite the cannula.

Extravasation (infiltration, tissuing)

This is the accidental infiltration of IV fluids/drugs into the SC tissue. It can cause local inflammation or pain. Mostly, there isn't a problem. However, tissue damage is more likely if the drug is hypertonic, chemically irritant or has a pH outside 4–8. The main culprits in this regard are:

- aciclovir, erythromycin, vancomycin

- calcium chloride, sodium bicarbonate

- dopamine and vasoactive agents

- phenobarbitone, phenytoin

- cytotoxic drugs

Index

Index

A

ACE inhibitors 8, 23, 25, 30
acid-peptic disorders 8–9, 90
acute confusion 40–2, 133
adenosine 65
administration
    frequency xi, 11, 106
    routes 10, 16–17, 123–4, 174,
      179, 218–20
adrenaline 173
alcohol abuse 43–7, 133, 144
alendronate 212
allergies xi, 206
allopurinol 28, 212
aminoglycosides 24, 28, 31, 32, 194–7
aminophylline 84, 200–2, 216–17
amiodarone 66, 67, 144, 174, 213–14
amoxicillin 28, 210
anaesthetics, local 118, 119
analgesia 5–6, 70, 72, 98, 105–20,
159–60
    see also NSAIDs; opioids
angina 60–3
anti-arrhythmics 64–7, 144, 197,
198–9, 213–14
anti-asthmatics 6, 13, 83–5, 200–2,
216–17
antibiotics 6, 13, 24, 90, 144, 161,
179–91
    see also specific drugs
anti-coagulants see heparin; warfarin
anti-convulsants 7–8, 14, 46, 72, 98,
126–30, 157–8
    see also carbamazepine; phenytoin
anti-depressants 9, 14
anti-emetics 7, 60, 63, 95–6, 110, 121,
123, 160–1
anti-fungals 8, 30, 31, 216
anti-histamines 7, 111, 205
anti-hypertensives 8, 23, 25
anti-Parkinsonian agents 157–8
anti-platelet agents 60, 156, 206–7
anti-viral agents 28, 31, 33
anxiolytics see benzodiazepines
APTT ratio 73, 149
ARBs (angiotensin receptor blockers)
8, 23
arrhythmia see anti-arrhythmics
aspirin 144, 206–7, 207–8
asthma 6, 13, 82, 83–5, 200–2, 206,
207–8, 216–17
atrial fibrillation (AF) 64–5, 139, 141
azathioprine 28, 91, 212

B

benzodiazepines 9, 42, 44–5, 127–8,
131, 133–6
beta-blockers 8, 13, 28, 32, 61, 66, 206
bisphosphonates 78, 212
blood pressure
    hypertension 8, 23, 25
    hypotension 66, 69, 118
    in SAH 69
bradycardia 118
breastfeeding 11–14
bronchodilators 6, 83–5

C

calcium 78, 80, 212, 213
calculations 26–7, 111–12, 122–3,
171–5, 196–7
carbamazepine 7, 203, 212–13, 215
cardiology 60–7, 197, 198–9
cellulitis 186
central venous lines 218–19
cephalosporins 6, 28–9, 206
charcoal 57
charts x–xiv, 119
children 15–19
chloral hydrate 29
chlordiazepoxide 44–5
chlormethiazole 45
chlorpromazine 42, 133, 134
cholestasis 97
ciclosporin 197, 203, 209, 211, 213,
215–16
ciprofloxacin 6, 29, 213, 216–17
cirrhosis 97
clarithromycin 29, 182, 212–13
clindamycin 29
Clostridium difficile 184, 185
co-amoxiclav 29
Cockcroft–Gault equation 27
co-codamol 30, 108–9
codeine 72, 107, 110, 160
co-dydramol 30, 108–9
colostomy 162
compliance xi, 18, 21–2
confusion, acute 40–2, 133
constipation see laxatives
contraindications 204–8
COPD 82–5, 183
corticosteroids 6, 10, 13, 71, 81, 85,
157, 176–8, 215
co-trimoxazole 30
COX-2 inhibitors 24, 205
creatinine clearance 26–7, 28–33
cyclizine 7, 96

D

DC cardioversion 64, 65, 66
deep vein thrombosis (DVT) 69, 139, 141, 147–51
delirium tremens 43–6
diabetes 34–9, 51–6, 61, 80, 163–5, 207
diamorphine 110, 111, 118, 123
diarrhoea 89–90, 184–5
diazepam 45, 127, 128, 133
diclofenac 6, 13, 107, 214–15
diet 26, 93, 143
digoxin 66, 197, 198–9, 213–14
dihydrocodeine 108, 110
discharging patients xiv, 21–2
diuretics 25, 63, 98, 214
documentation x–xiv, 17, 119, 145, 189
dyspepsia 8–9, 89
dyspnoea 82–5

E

elderly patients 20–2, 42, 128, 133, 142, 194
electrolytes 26, 52, 75–8, 80
empyema 182
endocarditis 187
epidural analgesia 117–20
epilepsy *see* anti-convulsants
erythromycin 30, 212–13, 216, 217
ethambutol 30

F

fentanyl 112–13, 118, 122
flucloxacillin 30
fluconazole 8, 30, 216
fluid replacement 51, 53, 70, 75, 158–9, 184
foetus, effects on 3–10
furosemide 63, 214

G

gabapentin 30
gastric ulcers 8–9, 90
gastroenteritis 184–5
gastrointestinal bleeding 90, 98
gentamicin 31, 194–7
glomerular filtration rate 27
glucagon 56
glucose–potassium–insulin infusions 36–7, 164
gravity flow administration 174

H

haloperidol 31, 96, 121
Hartford nomogram 196
headaches 70, 119
heart valve replacements 139, 141, 156
heparin 31, 69, 73

LMWH 6, 13, 61, 146–7, 148, 150–1
  unfractionated 7, 147–8, 149
hepatic disease 97–8, 205
hepatic enzymes 193, 209, 211
hydration 51, 53, 70, 75, 158–9, 184
hydrocortisone 81, 85, 215
hydroxyurea 31
hyperosmolar non-ketotic coma 53–4
hypertension 8, 23, 25
hyperthyroidism 78–9
hypnotics 29, 33, 131, 133–6
hypoglycaemia 55–6, 80
hypotension 66, 69, 118
hypothyroidism 31, 81

I

ibuprofen 6, 13, 107, 214–15
ileostomy 162
imipenem 31
immunosuppressants 157–8, 203, 209, 213, 215–16
inflammatory bowel disease 91
inhaled drugs 6, 17, 83
INR (international normalisation ratio) 98, 140–4
insomnia 131–6
insulin 34–8, 51, 54, 164, 165
interactions 142–5, 209–17
intravenous administration 17, 123–4, 174, 179, 218–20
intravenous contrast media 24
ipratropium bromide 83
isotretinoin 10
itraconazole 31, 216

J

jaundice 97
jejunostomy 162

K

ketoacidosis 51–2
kidney disease 23–33, 193, 205, 207

L

labetalol 13, 31
laxatives 9, 13, 69, 92–4, 98, 166–7
  with opioids 111, 121, 159
levomepromazine 96, 123
lithium 9, 14, 24, 203, 214–15
liver disease 97–8, 205
liver enzymes 193, 209, 211
LMWH (low molecular weight heparin) 6, 13, 61, 146–7, 148, 150–1
loperamide 162
lorazepam 42, 45, 127

M

macrolides 29, 30, 182, 212–13, 216, 217
magnesium 80
magnesium chloride 85
malnutrition 99–101
mannitol 71–2
meningitis 180–1
meropenem 31
metabolic emergencies 75–81
metformin 31, 39, 164, 165, 207
methadone 110, 215
methyldopa 8, 32
metoclopramide 96, 207
metronidazole 184
midazolam 127
misoprostol 8–9
morphine 32, 110, 111–12, 121–3, 205
MRSA infections 188, 189
myocardial infarction 60–3

N

NAC (N-acetyl cysteine) 57–9
naloxone 111
nasogastric feeds 215
nausea 95–6, 123, 160–1
    see also anti-emetics
nebulisation 83–4
necrotising fasciitis 186
neonatal withdrawal syndrome 5, 9
nephrotoxicity 23–5
neurosurgery 68–72, 148
neutropenic sepsis 188
nil by mouth 155–6
nimodipine 69
nitrates 31, 61, 63
nitrazepam 133, 134
NSAIDs 106, 107, 108
    side effects/interactions 144, 205, 207–8, 214–15
    specific patient groups 6, 13, 24, 72, 98

O

obesity 27, 146, 189, 196–7
oedema 25, 63–4
older patients 20–2, 42, 128, 133, 142, 194
ondansetron 96
opioids
    analgesia 106, 107–8, 109–13, 118, 159–60
    anti-diarrhoeal 90, 184
    calculations 111–12, 122–3, 171–2
    emergency prescribing 60, 63, 70, 72
    in palliative care 121–3
    specific patient groups 5, 14, 98, 205

toxicity 111, 122
oral hypoglycaemic agents 31, 39, 164, 165, 207
otitis media 181
oxygen therapy 42, 60, 63, 82

P

Pabrinex® 46–7
paediatrics 15–19
pain relief see analgesia; NSAIDs; opioids
palliative care 121–5
paracetamol 5, 106, 107, 109, 159
    overdose 57–9
patient-controlled analgesia 114–16
penicillins 6, 28, 30, 32, 206, 208
percentages 172–3
pharmacokinetics 20, 38, 97, 193, 205, 209–10, 211
pharyngitis 181
phenobarbitone 7, 129, 203, 213
phenytoin 7, 32, 128–9, 197, 199–200, 210, 213, 215
pneumonia 182–4
polypharmacy 20, 24, 124
potassium 76–7, 80
    in diabetes 36–7, 52, 53
PPIs (proton-pump inhibitors) 8, 90
prednisolone 10, 13, 85, 157, 177, 215
pregnancy 3–10, 187
procyclidine 42
promazine 133, 134
promethazine 7, 133, 134
protamine sulphate 147
pruritus 98, 111
pseudomembranous colitis 184, 185
pulmonary embolism (PE) 73–4, 139, 141, 147, 148
pulmonary oedema 63–4
pyrazinamide 32

Q

quinolones 6, 29, 213, 216–17

R

ratios 173
re-feeding syndrome 100
renal disease 23–33, 193, 205, 207
respiratory disease 82–5, 181–4
rifampicin 32, 209, 215

S

safety, basics x–xiv
salbutamol 6, 83, 84
sedation 40–2, 44–6, 131, 133–6
seizures 46, 126–30
    see also anti-convulsants
septicaemia 187–8
shock 63

simvastatin 215–16
skin diseases 10
sodium supplementation 80
splenectomy 161
SSRIs 9, 14
statins 26, 62, 215–16
status epilepticus 128–30
steroids *see* corticosteroids
stomas 162
subarachnoid haemorrhage 68–71
supraventricular tachycardia 65–6
surgery
    before 74, 155–8, 161, 163–4,
        166–7, 189–91
    after 114–16, 150–1, 158–61,
        162, 165
syringe drivers 123–4, 174

T

tacrolimus 216
tamoxifen 32
tazocin 32
teicoplanin 32
temazepam 9, 133, 134
teratogenesis 4, 6, 7, 8, 9, 10
tetracyclines 6, 32, 213
theophylline 84, 200–2, 216–17
therapeutic drug monitoring 192–203,
    211
thiamine 46–7
thrombolysis 61–3, 73–4
thyroid disease 31, 78–9, 81

topical drugs 5, 10
total parenteral nutrition 99–101
tramadol 32, 108, 112, 160
tricyclic anti-depressants 9, 14
trimethoprim 6, 33

U

units of measurement 171–2
urinary tract infections 186–7

V

valproate 7, 32, 203
vancomycin 33, 202
venlafaxine 33
ventricular tachycardia 66
verapamil 65, 214
vitamin B1 46–7
vitamin K 98, 142, 143
vomiting 95–6, 123, 160–1, 184–5
    see also anti-emetics

W

warfarin 7, 33, 71, 74, 139–45,
    156–7, 206–7
weight of patients xi, 196–7
Wernicke–Korsakoff syndrome 46
Wernicke's encephalopathy 46–7

Z

zopiclone 33, 131, 133